LOVE YOUR BREASTS

LOVE YOURSELF

A COMPREHENSIVE AND HOLISTIC APPROACH TO **BREAST CARE** INSIDE AND OUT

LILIAN O. EBUOMA MD

Copyright © 2024 Lilian O. Ebuoma, MD

All rights reserved. This book or parts thereof may not be reproduced in any form, stored in any retrieval system, or transmitted in any form by any means—electronic, mechanical, photocopy, recording, or otherwise—without prior written permission of the author, except as provided by United States of America copyright law.

ISBNs:
eBook	979-8-9916401-0-7
Paperback	979-8-9916401-1-4
Hardcover	979-8-9916401-2-1

Library of Congress Control Number: 2024920669

For image credits see page 227.

First Edition
Book Production by Hal Clifford Associates
www.hcabooks.com

By reading this document, the reader agrees that under no circumstances is the author or the publisher responsible for any losses, direct or indirect, which are incurred as a result of the use of information contained within this document, including, but not limited to, errors, omissions, or inaccuracies.

Legal Notice:

This book is copyright protected. Please note the information contained within this document is for educational and personal use only. You cannot amend, distribute, sell, use, quote or paraphrase any part, or the content within this book, without the consent of the author or publisher.

www.lilianebuoma.com
Cape Girardeau, Missouri 63701

DISCLAIMER

Medical information published in this book is strictly for informational purposes only and does not replace or preclude medical advice provided by licensed healthcare professionals, such as your doctor. Given the dynamic nature of the medical industry, we have made special considerations to ensure correctness, relevance, and completeness of the subject matter. Despite all the precautions, errors are possible, and information may also become outdated. The reader assumes full and sole responsibility for any action taken based on the information provided in this book. All the information presented should be carefully reviewed with your healthcare provider, and as such, neither the author, editor or other representatives of the publisher of this book, and its subsidiaries or others acting on behalf of the author is liable for any explicit, implicit, exceptional or otherwise harmful incidence.

This book and all components and elements thereof cannot be reproduced, duplicated, distributed, or modified in any form without explicit written permission from the author.

TABLE OF CONTENT

INTRODUCTION	1
SECTION 1. GETTING INTIMATE WITH YOUR BREASTS.	**9**
Chapter 1. The Meaning of Our Breasts	11
Chapter 2. The Biology of the Breast	19
SECTION 2. BREAST HEALTH 101: WHAT'S HEALTHY AND WHAT'S NOT?	**29**
Chapter 3. Common Breast Problems: Symptoms, Causes, and Treatment	31
Chapter 4. Breast Lumps: A Mini-Guide to the Different Types of Breast Masses	43
SECTION 3. BREAST CANCER: FACTS, DIAGNOSIS, TREATMENT, AND SURVIVORSHIP.	**51**
Chapter 5. Breast Cancer Facts	53
Chapter 6. Fear and Breast Cancer: You're Not Alone	61
Chapter 7. Breast Cancer Stigma and Myths	65
Chapter 8. Breast Cancer Risk Factors and Prevention	77
Chapter 9. Breast Cancer Prevention and Early Detection	85
Chapter 10. Breast Cancer Diagnosis and Treatment Journey	101
Chapter 11. Survivorship: Beyond the Diagnosis	109
Chapter 12. Love Your Breasts; Love Yourself	131
SECTION 4. DIET FOR BREAST HEALTH	**141**
BREAKFAST	145
LUNCH	157
DINNER	169
BEVERAGES	181
SNACKS	191
SECTION 5. FITNESS FOR OPTIMAL BREAST HEALTH	**197**
NOTES	213

EDUCATION IS THE MOST
POWERFUL WEAPON WHICH
YOU CAN USE TO CHANGE
THE WORLD.

—*NELSON MANDELA*

INTRODUCTION

OUR BREASTS UNIFY US AS WOMEN, MOTHERS, DAUGHTERS, and sisters. They are life-giving, shape-giving, a topic of conversation, and the subject of deep and changing meaning over time. Each woman has a different relationship with her breasts. For some, breasts symbolize their womanhood. For others, they are a biological marker of their ability to nurture a child. Some women believe their breasts are central to their sexual and individual identity, while others are indifferent about them. No matter how you feel about your breasts or what they mean to you, they are an essential part of your body.

Your breast health matters. You matter.

BREAST CANCER

Breast cancer is the most common female malignancy in the world. In 2021, Sung et al. reported that, based on GLOBOCAN 2020 estimates of cancer incidence and the mortality report produced by the IARC, breast cancer had surpassed lung cancer as the most common female malignancy in the world. A woman is diagnosed with breast cancer every fourteen seconds. A woman in America is diagnosed with breast cancer every two minutes. According to the American Cancer Society, there will be 287,850 new cases of invasive breast cancer and 43,250 deaths in women in the United States in 2022.

Yet so many women don't know the early signs of this disease, or how to monitor for it, or even understand their breasts well enough to notice if anything is abnormal. They are disempowered—and from such an essential aspect of their health.

Nor is this disempowerment evenly distributed; it divides along country and community lines. For example, a Black woman in the

United States, a high-income country, has a 20 percent to 40 percent mortality rate from breast cancer compared to a Caucasian woman. In a low-income country like Nigeria, the mortality rate from breast cancer is greater than 50 percent to 70 percent at five years. Contrast this with a greater than 90 percent survival rate in developed countries.

Sadly, some Black women do not have access to adequate information or healthcare regarding their breast health. This lack of access to life-saving information and healthcare access means Black women will continue to die prematurely from breast cancer. In the case of Black women in sub-Saharan Africa, the health facilities available for the preventive screening and diagnostic evaluation of breast cancer are few, limited in capacity, and of uncertain quality. Galukande et al. shed light on the mortality outcomes and the major intergenerational consequences associated with breast cancer deaths in sub-Saharan Africa. They found that for every 100 deaths in women younger than fifty, there were 210 maternal orphans. A 1:2 ratio! In the United States, Alsheik et al. found that compared to other races, Black women received fewer screening mammograms and were less likely to receive digital breast tomosynthesis (DBT), even though DBT has been shown to increase the cancer detection rate and decrease recall rates.

Sociocultural issues also serve as barriers to health-seeking behavior. There is a general distrust of the healthcare system in the Black community, and several research studies have shown a fatalistic perception of breast cancer. In addition, other attitudes and beliefs, such as stigmas in this population and other psychological barriers, lead to the delayed onset of routine breast cancer screening and delayed presentation for diagnosis and treatment of breast cancer.

Given the medical advancements in breast cancer treatment, I believe it should not be this way. I find it disheartening that despite the availability of vital information to improve the prognosis of breast cancer, it remains inaccessible to a large subset of women. When women are better educated and better equipped, they will act sooner. An informed woman can act sooner when she notices a change in her breasts or is told of a new change or suspicious findings after her routine screening, thereby taking advantage of early detection.

This is why I wrote this book—because the first step to bridging disparity and shaping a path to empowerment is education.

THIS BOOK IS FOR YOU

My grandmother was a midwife, one of the first to be trained in Nigeria. She always said to me, "Never be idle when there is pain and suffering in this world." When I chose to pursue radiology at Harvard Medical School, I chose breast imaging as a sub-specialization because I knew it had impact beyond clinical and interpretative skills—it had the potential to make an extensive difference. Since then, I've been on a quest to change the status quo: to educate women about breast cancer so as to decrease mortality and morbidity rates, especially among disadvantaged communities, and to empower women to take charge of their health and their lives.

Questions and concerns from women from various walks of life, with different beliefs, attitudes, and challenges regarding breast health, inspired this book. I wrote it for every woman who wants to take charge of her breast health and shape her own journey.

You may be the woman having sleepless nights because you believe your recurring breast pain is due to cancer.

You may be the mother of four with a breast lump that has been pushing into your skin for two years now but who is afraid to face a cancer diagnosis.

You may be the woman avoiding a screening mammogram because you are petrified of the "C" word and believe no news is good news.

You may be the woman concerned about the changes you have seen in your breasts but don't know who to turn to or where to get the proper care.

You may be the woman who is aware of the negative impact a lack of knowledge and awareness can have on your health, and you are choosing to learn more.

No matter your situation, this book is for you. By gaining a greater holistic understanding of the biological purpose and significance of the breasts, as well as knowledge about how to care for your breasts, you are empowering yourself to love and accept your body as it changes throughout the different stages of life, and to act fast when abnormal changes take place.

As the president and founder of the Lily Cares Foundation, an NGO focused on empowering women, and the founder of Lilly Women's Health Breast Care Center, a comprehensive breast care and imaging facility in Nigeria, I've seen firsthand what it is like when women don't have access to information that empowers them, and when the systems and the society around them leave them behind. I want to change that; I want to reach out to those who are visibly invisible, who are discarded or erased; I want them to know that someone is paying attention. All women deserve access to quality healthcare and information regardless of who they are and where they live in the world. This book intends to bring empowering information closer to you. It is not a substitute for medical advice, but after reading this book, you will be better equipped to take charge of your breast health. You will know what is considered healthy and when to seek medical attention.

In addition to knowing and understanding more about your breast health, I want you to think about yourself. *Yes, you!* Your relationship with yourself, mindset, limiting beliefs, and what has influenced your thinking. You are magnificent, fearfully and wonderfully made! Are you honoring yourself and your values? How much value do you place on your self-worth? And are you demanding it from yourself and others?

My ultimate desire is to provide you with the tools for optimal living, so that you can move toward being the truest and highest version of yourself. You deserve to "be" because "you are."

Be visible! Keep on living!
LILIAN O. EBUOMA, MD

This book is dedicated to my grandma Alice, aka "Mummy Adepegba," who taught me to never be idle when there is pain and suffering.

To help you easily navigate the information in this book, I have divided it into the following five sections:

Section 1: Getting Intimate with Your Breasts. A critical look at the history of how humans have seen women's breasts in history and what they have meant to different societies.

Section 2: Breast Health 101: What's Healthy and What's Not? The most common breast problems and corresponding treatment.

Section 3: Breast Cancer: Facts, Diagnosis, Treatment, and Survivorship. The epidemiology of breast cancers looking at the incidence, prevalence, and survival rate for symptomatic and screen-detected breast cancers. Diagnosis, treatment, and beyond.

Section 4: Diet for Breast Health. Simple recipes and a meal plan to boost breast health the easy, natural, and delicious way.

Section 5: Fitness for Optimal Breast Health. Easy workout plan for breast and general health enhancement.

SECTION 1
GETTING INTIMATE WITH YOUR BREASTS.

A critical look at the history of how humans have seen women's breasts in history and what they have meant to different societies.

CHAPTER 1
THE MEANING OF OUR BREASTS

MUCH ADO ABOUT BREASTS: SYMBOLISM OF THE BREASTS

Ah, breasts. Perky, flat, too big, too small . . . the list of how we analyze, criticize, and elevate the breasts goes on and on. Lucky is the woman who has a set that she's perfectly happy with.

No matter how we feel about our breasts, they are a symbol of womanhood; breasts have much value and meaning not just to the woman who holds them, but also to the rest of humankind.

They're stared at and admired. They're chuckled at and hidden from view. Today, they're regarded as the ultimate symbol of female sexuality, when not too long ago, they were a symbol of the ability to nurture a child. And they've had hundreds of other meanings along the way.

This chapter explores the many representations of female breasts over the centuries.

WHY DO WE CARE SO MUCH ABOUT BREASTS?

From a biological perspective, breasts have the primary function of providing a food source for infants. However, they get attention for, well, just being breasts. Our society today has a deep-rooted fascination and preoccupation with the female breasts. Glance up at a billboard advertising clothing, turn on the TV, scroll through social media, or take a walk down the street—no matter where you look, they are everywhere!

Why is this, and when did this transition take place from nurture to sex symbol? We can begin to unlock the answer by looking at some of the most fascinating milestones in human breast history.

SOURCE OF SUSTENANCE AND LIFEFORCE

Breasts have always symbolized power, but their earliest power was not sexually focused. In fact, breasts were anything *but* sexual, with breasts regarded as a nurturing, life-giving force. The ancient Egyptians held this view way back around 3000 B.C., as evidenced by depictions of the Egyptian goddess Isis. This goddess of nature and fertility is shown breastfeeding her son Horus, giving him the needed nourishment to thrive.

Christianity kept up this tradition of breasts as a nurturing force throughout the thirteenth and fourteenth centuries, with plenty of depictions of the Virgin Mary breastfeeding baby Jesus. The Virgin Mother's breast is clearly exposed in many of these religious paintings, performing a function regarded as natural and even beautiful.

Breasts provided food for the body on a literal level and food for the soul on a symbolic one. The primary function of breasts is to feed and sustain life—at the most basic level, that is what they are built for. An infant's first source of sustenance is his mother's milk—the most nourishing of foods. In addition to nutrition, the first meaningful physical contact outside of the womb, which promotes bonding, is at the breasts. When a child is at her mother's bosom, suckling milk is the first feeling of love, warmth, and trust they experience. At the same time, breastfeeding triggers the production of oxytocin (the love hormone), which helps build a strong bond between mother and baby.

BREASTS AS MOTHER EARTH

Drawing on the breasts' innate ability to nurture and sustain life, many thinkers have considered them a symbol of nature itself. In the words of writer Laura Hamilton, "Fertile mounds of earth, majestic mountains, nurturing waters, all relate to the shape and function of breasts." Hamilton likens the hills to a "rounded bosom of a woman, while the flow of rivers or water coincides with a mother's milk." In this sense, breasts become a representation of the gorgeous glory of Mother Earth. With their prime location near the heart, breasts can also symbolize love. This view again shifts back to spiritual traditions that focused on the sacred values of love, wisdom, and compassion that burst from the heart of a woman.

BREASTS AS FORBIDDEN PLEASURE

The so-called "secularization of the breast" occurred when the breast lost its sacred, symbolic power and began to be viewed in the sexual sense.

Author Margaret Miles gets credit for coining the term in her book *A Complex Delight: The Secularization of the Breast*. The shift can largely be attributed to the rise of the printing press, which provided tons of information from authorities other than the church.

This led to a split view of the female body as a source of either *good* or *evil*. The positive depictions pointed to the Virgin Mary and the female saints, while the "evil" depictions were flooded with imagery of the sexual temptresses. The breast, likewise, went from the life-giving, nurturing symbol to one of sin and forbidden pleasure.

BREASTS AND SEXUALITY

Once the seventeenth century swept in, pornography came right along with it. Medical books depicting the female body in detail were already circulating, and the printing press made it easy to distribute illustrated pornographic literature to the world at large.

Thus, the female breast became firmly entrenched as a sexual object, a far cry from its previous status as a symbol of nourishment and life. This sexual view of breasts remains the norm today and is one of the reasons breastfeeding in public makes some people uncomfortable. They just can't shake the idea of the breast as an erotic object. (States like Indiana and Michigan regard showing of the female breast with less than a fully opaque covering of any part of the nipple a crime!

In Louisiana, female breast nipples exposed with the intent of sexual arousal is also a no-no.)

THE SYMBOL OF WOMANHOOD

What clearly separates a woman from a man, at first glance, is the often-noticeable rise of the chest, thanks to the existence of breasts. In a sociocultural and anthropological light, larger breasts denote a healthier woman who is more readily able to nurture a child. This is because people think that voluminous breasts are an indication of a woman's ability to produce more milk, and therefore a greater capacity to provide sustenance to children. Of course, we now know that breast size has nothing to do with a woman's ability to produce milk.

For feminists, the breast is also often utilized as a symbol of empowerment, in response to a society that covered up and *controlled* breasts through garments—actions they feel subjugate or oppress women. In protests from women activist groups it is not uncommon to see members unclothe themselves to display their breasts. The public exposure hopes to send the clear message that a woman's body should be freed from oppression, whether it is through perceived oppressive instruments (clothing or constraints) or societal rules (disallowing or controlling how breastfeeding is done in public, for example).

THE BRA EVOLUTION

While most women today wouldn't dare leave the house without wearing a bra, the handy-dandy undergarment is a relatively modern invention. Ancient Egyptian women would be bare breasted beneath their loose, flowing tunics. The ancient Romans didn't have bras, either, although they did have a contraption known as the "breast band" or fascia. Young girls wore them to prevent their breasts from "sagging" in their later years.

Even more support came around in the sixteenth century with the invention of the tightly binding corset. Aristocratic women were the first to wear these stifling undergarments that shaped their waistlines and pushed up their breasts to unnatural proportions.

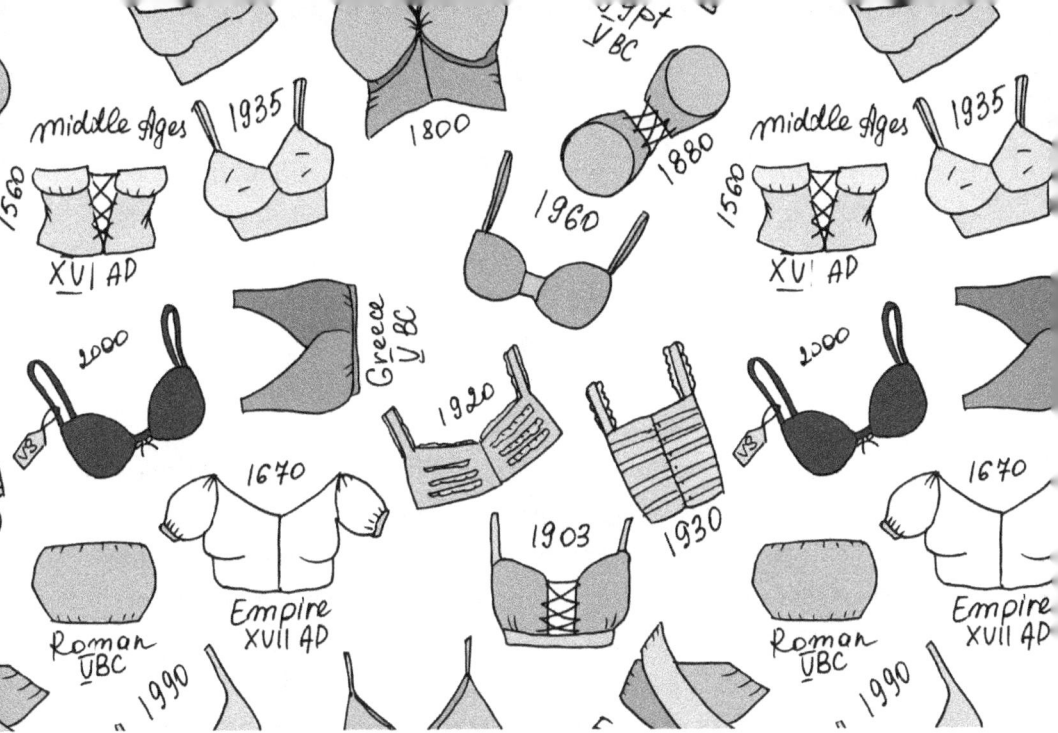

The corset reigned supreme for the next four hundred years or so until a Frenchwoman named Herminie Cadolle had the bright idea of dividing the corset into two separate garments in 1869. The top half became the modern bra in France she named "corselet-gorge."

The bra officially emerged in America in 1893, with the first US bra patent filed by Marie Tucek. While her design is essentially the same one used in today's underwire bras, Tucek's bra was a flop due to a lack of effective marketing. Throughout the early twentieth century, though, there were significant developments in bra design and technology. The word "brassiere" first appeared in American Vogue in 1907. By 1911, it was part of the Oxford English dictionary. Still, the corset continued to be the undergarment of choice for women.

Somewhere around 1910, New York City socialite Mary Phelps Jacobs couldn't stand how her whalebone corset looked under her sheer evening gown. So, the nineteen-year-old created a "backless brassiere" out of two handkerchiefs and pink silk ribbon. It became the most widely used bra design, and she eventually sold her patent to the Warner Brothers Corset Company.

America finally gave up on the corset around 1918, at the end of World War I. The corset was too impractical for women entering the workforce. Besides, a metal shortage made the steel used in corsets a hot commodity. The brassiere became the undergarment of choice.

In the 1920s, the bandeau bra and cup sizes emerged. The former flattened women's breasts so they could wear their straight-cut flapper dresses. The latter accentuated the breasts rather than flattening them. Cup sizes came about through a collaboration of Maidenform founders Ida and William Rosenthal, along with Enid Bissett.

The 1930s saw a trade of the old-school word "brassiere" for the fashionable, modern-day "bra." It also saw the assignment of cup sizes from the S. H. Camp and Company, which sized them from A through D.

World War II gave rise to undergarment styles like the torpedo bra, and a British survey found the average woman owned 1.2 bras by 1941. The later 1940s and 1950s saw the invention of the first padded bra, the push-up bra, and the front-hook bra. Credit for all three goes to Frederick Mellinger, the guy behind Frederick's of Hollywood. Sweater girls Marilyn Monroe and Lana Turner helped popularize the bullet bra, which gave the appearance of a larger cup size. The 1950s Baby Boom gave rise to maternity bras and starter bras for teens and preteens.

Four hundred women threw their bras in a trash can in 1968 as part of a protest of the Miss America pageant. While they wanted to burn these *instruments of female torture*, the cops wouldn't let them. But the "bra burners" moniker stuck.

The first sports bra, known then as the "Jogbra," hit the scene in 1977. It was created by three women who first got the idea by using two jockstraps. This was the same year Victoria's Secret made its debut. The cone bra made headlines in 1990 when Madonna wore the Jean Paul Gaultier design during her Blond Ambition tour. Bras got even wilder by 1996, when the fantasy bra was launched at Victoria Secret fashion shows.

By 2009, it was found that the average woman owned sixteen bras at any given time. Four million bras are manufactured per day!

Additional developments in the bra industry over recent years include a memory-foam bra, an anti-wrinkle bra, and a new range of cup sizes, reaching as high as an N cup. The average woman in the United States wears a 34DD. Interestingly, over 75 percent of women wear the wrong bra size—it just goes to show how little we end up knowing about our own breasts and how to dress them.

The most elaborate fantasy bra yet is a $12.5 million, gem-encrusted bra set in 18-karat gold.

WHAT DOES IT ALL MEAN FOR YOUR HEALTH?

The female breasts are a powerful life-giving force, and they are as essential as other parts of the body. The awareness of breasts usually starts at puberty for most girls around the age of ten to thirteen. During pregnancy and lactation, women are encouraged to nourish their bodies to have an adequate and nutrient-packed milk supply to feed their infants. Whether one is a mother or not, all women are encouraged to act differently when specific changes arise in their breasts.

Different factors account for some of the changes a woman may notice in her breasts, such as age, hormone status, medications, breastfeeding, and others. These changes may cause pain, lumps, skin irritation, discharge, clogged ducts, infection, and cancer. The most important signs to monitor are those that could indicate breast cancer, which can be fatal if not treated early and adequately.

MAIN TAKEAWAYS

Ultimately, all these different levels of meanings are attributed to the general idea that breasts are a *source of power*. Breasts can provide nourishment to sustain life, indicate empowerment as a woman in a way that a man cannot, and captivate (or even to some extent, manipulate) the opposite sex by adding breasts to a woman's come-hither projection.

As you can see, there are so many ideas about the female breasts that are tied to their functional and symbolic meanings for humanity throughout history.

Breasts are a symbol of femininity and womanhood, and being a woman means possessing the following values: compassion, love, and wisdom—all fundamental values that, when cultivated, nurtured, and passed on, lead to better and more loving individuals who make up society.

CHAPTER 2
THE BIOLOGY OF THE BREAST

*Good evening. Please, how can one enlarge
or reduce her breast size?*
—Anonymous

AN INTRODUCTION TO BREAST DEVELOPMENT

Breasts begin to develop during the gestational period while the baby is still in the mother's womb. At this stage, the breasts begin to form as two lines called "mammary ridges," which extend from the armpit area to the lower abdomen/thigh. These two lines regress as the baby develops, and only the cells in the chest area remain.

Sometimes parts of the cells along the mammary ridge can remain in areas other than the chest. This can result in having actual accessory breast tissue in the armpit (the medical term for which is "polymastia or supernumerary breast tissue") or even an extra nipple on the belly! Some women only become aware of an accessory breast tissue when they notice tenderness or a lump in the armpit area or even breastmilk oozing out of their abdomen or thigh during lactation!

The breasts continue to develop and change as a girl matures.

There are five stages of breast growth, but it is vital to keep in mind that everyone is different, so development, size, and shape vary.

Stages of breast development

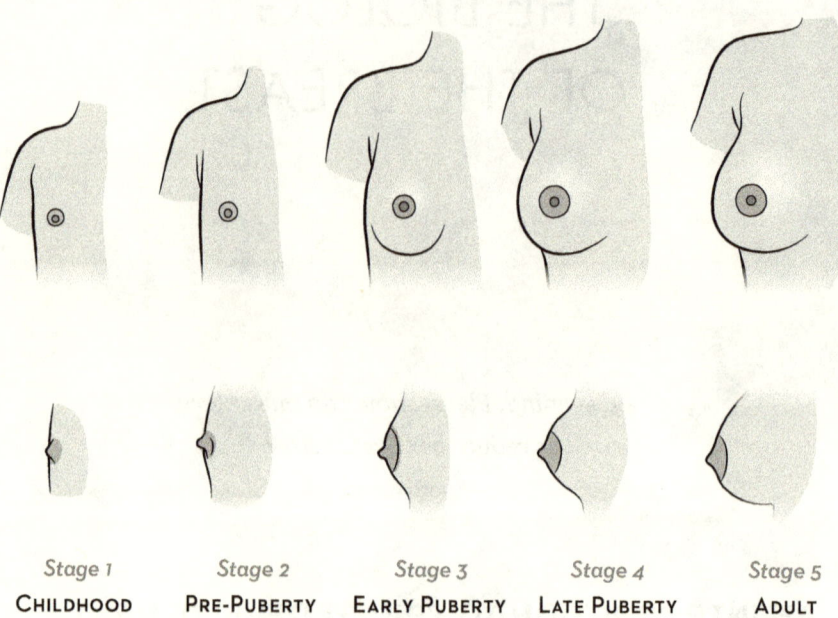

Stage 1 — CHILDHOOD
Stage 2 — PRE-PUBERTY
Stage 3 — EARLY PUBERTY
Stage 4 — LATE PUBERTY
Stage 5 — ADULT

- **Stage 1: Childhood.** This is the stage before puberty. During this stage, the breasts are flat and have not yet begun to develop, and the nipples are only slightly raised.
  The breasts typically begin to develop during this stage, which is usually around the age of seven or eight but may be as late as fourteen. There is a flat, small bud that develops under the nipples, which causes the nipple (the pointy part of your breast) to stick out from the chest while the areola (the darker area around the nipple) gets larger. These buds contain tissue, fat, and milk glands.
- **Stage 2: Early Puberty.** During this stage, the breasts become bigger, and the areolas continue to grow larger. A girl is usually ten to thirteen years old at this stage, but it may occur in girls as young as ten or older than thirteen. This stage may last for a few months to about two years.

- **Stage 3: Late Puberty**. The nipple and areola continue to grow bigger during this stage. They also separate to form a small mound on the breast. It is at this stage that the breasts often have a cone or pointed shape. This stage usually occurs in girls aged twelve to fourteen, and it typically lasts from about eight months to two years.
- **Stage 4: Mature Breast Stage**. The nipple and areola continue to grow bigger during this stage. They also separate to form a more defined breast mound, with the areola and nipple forming a raised secondary mound on top. During this stage, the breasts often have a cone or pointed shape. This stage typically occurs during late puberty or early adulthood. It's important to remember that every individual's development timeline is unique, and factors such as genetics, hormones, and overall health can influence the onset and progression of breast development.
- **Stage 5: Adult**. This is the adult stage. The areola and nipple are no longer a separate mound from the breast. The breasts are usually fully developed by the end of stage 5, which typically occurs during the ages of thirteen to sixteen.

A note about inverted nipple: Sometimes, after breasts are fully developed, some women may have nipples that point inward; this is totally normal. However, if you've always had protruded nipples and they suddenly point inward, you should see your doctor to make sure there isn't a lump in your breast that is pulling it inward.

BREAST SIZE

One of the most common concerns and complaints I hear from women is related to the size of their breasts. Honestly, it's hard not to think about how our breasts stack up against others'.

Models and celebrities with *perfect* breasts and bodies are flaunted about all day long on TV, magazines, and social media. Women with small breasts often feel as though they don't look like the women on the cover of magazines, or they don't feel as attractive as their friends with larger breasts. Young girls and teenagers often feel their breasts attract too much attention as they develop. Ladies with large breasts often complain of them being heavy and causing shoulder and back pain.

You may have concerns no matter the size or shape of your breasts, but it is essential to know that all women have unique breasts, and no size or shape is healthier than the next.

If you're curious about how your breasts got to be the size and shape they are, we can have a look at many factors: nutrition, weight, hormonal status, age. But the major determinant of breast size, which can't be changed, is your DNA. That's right, your parents!

LARGE OR SMALL, GOD MADE THEM ALL

Women can have a variety of feelings when it comes to the size and shape of their breasts. The size of the breast can influence self-confidence when it is associated with attraction and sexuality. On the other hand, if you are uncomfortable with your physical appearance, it may influence your happiness and satisfaction with life in general.

The belief that breast size affects interpersonal and social relations is common for women of all ages, especially teenagers and young adults. At some point in life, most women have experienced concerns related to the size of their breasts. For example, when out in public, women with either large or very small breasts can become self-conscious. Also, it can be difficult for women with large breasts to find well-fitting clothes that suit their fashion sense and the occasion. At the same time, women with small breasts may find it hard to choose clothes that flatter their figure.

The truth is the different shapes and sizes of breasts appeal to different types of people. Media propaganda aside, who really determines the perfect breasts? Anyone! Women can and should be comfortable with their bodies regardless of their breast size. After all, you've been fearfully and wonderfully made by your Creator.

However, if the size of your breasts has a significant impact on your happiness, quality of life, and/or health, there are several options available to help you modify the size and/or shape of your breasts.

PETITE BREASTS: WHAT TO DO ABOUT IT?

Breast size is determined by a combination of genetics, lifestyle, and body weight. Below are some non-surgical reasons the breast size may increase or appear larger.

- **Weight Gain**. Breast tissue consists of fatty and fibrous tissue. Therefore, weight gain can make your breasts larger. Improving your diet may help you gain weight in your breasts, especially if you are underweight. However, increasing your calories (amount of food you eat) if you are currently at an ideal weight or overweight can cause you to gain more pounds in less desirable places, such as your belly! So be careful.
- **Hormones**. The two primary female hormones are estrogen and progesterone. Some birth control pills, which can have different combinations of the two female hormones, may cause an unintended increase in breast size in certain women. You may also be able to increase your breast size with the use of estrogen creams. I personally do not endorse the use of exogenous estrogen (i.e., estrogen that is not made inside your body) unless medically indicated due to the high risk of unintended health consequences. It is essential that you talk with your doctor before considering this method, as many medical professionals agree that an excessively high level of estrogen may be linked to certain cancers.
- **Exercise**. Working out your pectoral muscles (the muscles under your breasts) may lift your breasts outward and make them look and appear larger. See workout routines in **Section 5: Fitness for Optimal Breast Health.**

Non-surgical solutions are temporary measures and will not result in extreme or significant change in breast size. If you are keen on increasing your bust size, surgery is typically the most definitive way to do it.

Surgical Solutions: Breast Augmentation Surgery

Surgical augmentation to increase size, reconstruction after surgery, or correcting development defects can be done with implants using a medical device (implant) or a fat transfer. According to the 2020 International Society of Aesthetic Plastic Surgery (ISAPS) survey, breast augmentation is the most popular surgical cosmetic procedure in women globally, accounting for 16 percent of all surgical cosmetic procedures. It surpasses liposuction, a close second, which makes up 15 percent of all surgical cosmetic procedures. Younger women seeking breast augmentation surgery are typically looking to increase the volume of naturally small breasts. Older women seek augmentation to restore volume loss that can occur with age, childbirth, and breastfeeding.

The first breast augmentation was performed in Heidelberg, Germany, by Dr. Vicenz Czerny, the "father of plastic surgery," in 1895 by transplanting fat from the patient's thigh to a partial mastectomy site. The era of modern breast augmentation was ushered in by two plastic surgeons based in Houston, Texas, Dr. Thomas Cronin and Dr. Frank Gerow, with a silicone-based breast implant placement in 1962. Regulation of silicone by the Food and Drug Administration (FDA) began in 1976.

A moratorium was placed on silicone implants in the United States between 1992 and 2006 due to public concern and a lack of safety data. In 1998, Dow Corning, a company that manufactured silicone implants, agreed to pay $3.2 billion to settle a class action lawsuit by over 150,000 women who claimed the silicone implants made them ill. In 2006, after several studies showed that silicone implants did not cause breast cancer, connective tissue disorder, and other harmful illnesses, the moratorium was lifted.

In 1964, the company Laboroatoire Arion in France developed the first saline breast implant, with a silicone outer shell and saline-filled inner shell. Many types of breast implants are available today with different shapes, textures, fills, etc. The two main implant fillers are saline (salt water) and silicone.

Cosmetic breast implant surgery is typically performed after the age of eighteen. The FDA recommends saline implants for eighteen years and older, and silicone implants for twenty-two years and older.

Implants are placed under moderate or general anesthesia through a periareolar (around the nipple), inframammary fold (underneath the breast), or axillary (armpit). The implant can be placed in a **prepectoral** location between the chest muscles and the breast tissue, or in a **retropectoral** location, behind the muscle.

Risks vs. Benefits of Breast Augmentation Surgery

Like any surgery and especially with the implantation of a medical device, breast implant placement has associated risks. These are, but are not limited to, infection, pain, damage to your body, implant complications (rupture, contracture, leaks), and the possible need for more surgery. It is crucial to weigh the risks versus the benefits.

Suppose you do decide to go this route. In that case, I cannot stress the importance of choosing a doctor with ample experience with this procedure and an excellent safety record. Also, note that this is typically a costly procedure not covered by most insurance plans in the case of elective augmentation.

A Note about Augmentation with Free-Silicone Injections

Due to the high cost of breast implant surgery, some women may entertain the idea of injecting free silicone into their breasts. This is not the standard of care for augmentation, reconstruction, or body contouring. Its usage is strongly discouraged by the medical community and is typically done in a home setting by inexperienced and unlicensed individuals. In addition to the disfigurement that may occur, you cannot adequately verify what is being injected into your body, as non-medical-grade free silicone or other unknown substances sometimes may be used.

Although some may swear it is okay to inject free silicone into the breast based on the outward appearance, the inward effects can be catastrophic and possibly fatal. For instance, free silicone can migrate to a different area of the body than intended, the worst possible of which is the vascular system. Large amounts of free silicone can occlude blood vessels that return blood to your heart and have a similar effect as a blood clot (pulmonary embolus). Consider safer augmentation alternatives.

Breastfeeding and Breast Augmentation

Having breast implants may or may not affect one's ability to breastfeed in the future. During the surgery, milk glands and other breast structures may be injured, and this may interfere with breastfeeding. For instance, if the nerves are damaged, the letdown reflex may not function properly. Damage to the milk ducts may affect the flow of milk, and damage to the milk glands may decrease the amount of milk you can produce. There is also concern that silicone from implants can seep into breast milk. However, according to the Centers for Disease Control and Prevention (CDC), there is insufficient evidence to classify silicone implants as a contraindication to breastfeeding.

Silicone Implant Surveillance

A rare type of non-Hodgkin's lymphoma called breast implant-associated anaplastic large cell lymphoma (BIA-ALCL) has been associated with silicone breast implants. It is recommended that a non-contrast breast MRI be obtained three years after the initial surgery and every two years after that for surveillance.

Large Breasts: What to Do about It?

While some women with small breasts yearn to have large ones for various reasons like improved confidence, the opposite is also true. There are women with large breasts who want to have smaller breasts. This is typically due to some of the health and physical problems that large breasts may cause. For example, back pain is common in women with large breasts. The weight pulls the spine forward, creating postural challenges that put stress on the spine and back muscles. The shoulder muscles also work extra hard to carry the weight of the chest, which can lead to neck, shoulder, and back pain. Impingement of the nerves due to improper alignment and weight distribution of the neck, back, and shoulders can sometimes cause numbness and a tingling feeling in the arms and hands.

Non-Surgical Solutions

There aren't too many non-surgical solutions to reduce breast size, especially when the reason for wanting to reduce the breast is mainly for health purposes.

- **Weight loss:** Since breasts are made of fat, healthy weight loss might help some large-breasted women reduce a few sizes.
- **Supportive bras:** Wearing a supportive bra, such a sports bra, goes a long way toward helping alleviate neck, back, and shoulder symptoms.

Surgical Solutions: Breast Reduction Mammoplasty

Many women opt for breast reduction surgery for both medical and cosmetic reasons. If you have large breasts and are searching for the best way to reduce them, there are a few different options you can choose from, including the following:

- **Liposuction:** A procedure used to remove excess fat. This type of procedure is not suitable for all women; it is typically best for women who are overweight with excessive fatty tissue in their breasts.
- **Breast reduction surgery**: A procedure done under general anesthesia. The surgery is done to remove large volumes of breast tissue. Breast reduction surgery is the most common way to reduce breast size, and it can be life-changing for women with excessively large breasts. According to the 2020 International Society of

Aesthetic Plastic Surgery survey, it is the eighth most common surgical cosmetic surgery in the world. It is essential to do your homework and talk to more than one plastic surgeon, get all the facts regarding the surgery, and always verify the credentials of the surgeon you are considering.

Sagging or Drooping Breasts

Often women complain of sagging or droopy breasts after they have breastfed children or as they get older. Some women who are young and have not breastfed can also have droopy breasts due to their genetic makeup. Some of the non-surgical techniques that women with small breasts use include chest exercises, padded bras, or bra inserts. Women with this issue can also opt for a surgical procedure called a "mastopexy," which is a fancy name for a breast lift. The 2020 International Society of Aesthetic Plastic Surgery survey puts a breast lift as the sixth most common surgical cosmetic procedure in the world.

MAIN TAKEAWAYS

It is crucial to keep in mind that if you are a teenager or a young adult, your breasts will continue to grow and change. If you are older, changes associated with weight gain or loss, pregnancy, breastfeeding, and age-related factors will generally influence your breasts. Whether you are considering breast enlargement surgery, breast reduction surgery, or a breast lift, always discuss your options openly and honestly with a licensed plastic surgeon, and verify their qualifications through professional organizations, such as the American Academy of Cosmetic Surgery. Seek out others who have had the procedure, and get their honest opinion and feedback.

SECTION 2

BREAST HEALTH 101: WHAT'S HEALTHY AND WHAT'S NOT?

The most common breast problems and corresponding treatment.

CHAPTER 3
COMMON BREAST PROBLEMS: SYMPTOMS, CAUSES, AND TREATMENT

IN THIS CHAPTER, WE WILL focus on the prevention, detection, and treatment of breast diseases. "Senology" is the medical discipline that focuses on the study of benign and malignant breast diseases. Concerns that women have about their breast health include pain, palpable lumps, nipple discharge, fullness, etc. These concerns occur in women of all ages, from adolescents to the elderly. Most women fear that any breast symptom is a sign of breast cancer. Although discovering a problem with your breasts can be frightening, it is vital to keep in mind that most breast problems are benign and are not caused by breast cancer.

BREAST PAIN AND TENDERNESS

Breast pain, "mastalgia," is the most common breast symptom for which women seek the consultation of a healthcare professional. There are many reasons that a woman seeks care for breast pain, including "idiopathic" (i.e., when no underlying reason can be identified). Breast pain is more common in younger women and is typically a sign of a benign breast condition; it rarely indicates breast cancer. However, it is crucial to mention it to your healthcare provider to rule out any potential suspicious findings.

Breast pain can range from mild to severe enough that even a light touch or clothing can be bothersome. The pain can be intermittent or constant, and women can feel burning, throbbing, or tightness, or the area may be tender to touch. For some women, it can diminish their quality of life.

How Can You Know if Breast Pain Is Normal?

One way is to notice when you've felt similar pain in the past. If you feel pain in your breasts around the time of your period, for example, it is called cyclical breast pain. If the pain is irregular and not linked to your menstrual cycle, it is called non-cyclical breast pain. I go into further detail about each type of pain below so you can have a better understanding of each.

Cyclical Breast Pain

- Cyclical breast pain is related to your menstrual cycle and the changing balance between the two main female hormones—estrogen and progesterone. The increase in progesterone between when you ovulate and when you get your period (called the luteal phase, usually around the fourteenth to twenty-sixth days of a twenty-eight-day cycle) can make your breasts swell and feel full. They may sometimes become painful or tender.
- This type of breast pain typically affects both breasts, especially in the upper, outer area, though it may radiate to your underarms.
- It is usually accompanied by lumpiness and/or breast swelling.
- The feeling intensifies for two weeks before starting your period and eases up after the start of your period.
- It is more likely to affect women in their twenties to thirties but may affect women in their forties who are transitioning into menopause.

Non-Cyclical Breast Pain

- Non-cyclical breast pain is unrelated to your menstrual cycle.
- It typically affects women after menopause.
- It usually affects only one breast and is localized to one area, but it may spread across the breast.

For most women, breast pain resolves itself over time and may not need any treatment. However, you should see your doctor if the breast pain persists for longer than a couple of weeks, is getting progressively worse, interferes with daily activities, or occurs in one specific area of the breast.

Special Cases of Breast Pain

Pregnancy, breastfeeding, and menopause are also accompanied by hormonal changes that can cause breast pain. In general, these are considered normal, though they may be uncomfortable. Finding a bra that supports your breasts comfortably and adequately can help ease discomfort.

Non-Breast Related Pain

You may be experiencing pain that is not related to your breast but that instead affects the surrounding structures around the breast—for example:

- Muscle pain from the muscles of the ribs and upper body
- Pain in your ribs (trauma, arthritis, exercise, etc.)
- Acid reflux from the stomach
- Heart disease: Some women describe pain from their chest that travels to their arms. I always caution ladies not to forget about their heart health, especially when the breast has been cleared by your doctor and if the pain gets worse with activity.

Important!
Breast pain accompanied by a lump, bloody nipple discharge, skin dimpling, nipple retraction, and other suspicious signs and symptoms is concerning for cancer, and the pain should be considered as a secondary symptom. Medical and imaging evaluations should be performed immediately.

Seek medical attention immediately for pain that is in the chest, radiates to the arm, shoulder, or back, or worsens with activity. These may be signs of a heart attack.

BREAST PAIN REMEDIES

Breast pain is usually a self-limited condition and subsides without intervention. Remedies for breast pain range from avoidance of aggravating factors such as caffeinated products to prescription medications.

If you are concerned about your breast pain, it is best to see your doctor for a history and physical exam. Typically, if you are under thirty years old, your doctor will recommend a breast ultrasound scan. If you are over thirty, a mammogram will be performed to see if there are any abnormalities in the breast causing the pain.

If the pain persists, your doctor may prescribe non-sedating analgesics such as acetaminophen or nonsteroidal anti-inflammatory medications such as Ibuprofen. I have had patients who swear by evening primrose oil and Vitamin E oil in improving their breast pain symptoms. Prescription drugs such as gamolenic acid and bromocriptine have been studied in the use of breast pain. I strongly advise not to take any of these medicines except under the supervision of a trained medical practitioner. This is especially true when a woman is pregnant or breastfeeding.

> **Do not self-medicate.** Taking certain seemingly harmless medications in large quantities and without proper medical advice can interfere with other medications and cause ulcers, liver or kidney failure, and other potential deleterious effects.

One of the steps you can take to help ease the pain is to wear a comfortable bra that keeps the breasts as still as possible. Keep in mind that your breasts change size throughout your life, so making sure that your bra fits properly will help keep you comfortable.

Breast pain is usually a sign of a benign breast condition; it rarely indicates breast cancer. However, it is essential to get it evaluated to exclude breast cancer.

Nipple Discharge

The breast is made up of a system of lobules and ducts. About fifteen to twenty lactiferous ducts (milk ducts), which bring milk from the breast glands, converge centrally into the nipple, where milk is secreted. "Nipple discharge" refers to any fluid that comes out of the nipple of your breasts. **The breast is a modified sweat gland that contains ducts that secrete fluid.** Breast ducts, like other ducts in your body, have secretions, so it is not unusual to be able to squeeze out fluid that can be yellow, green, clear, or milky. In most situations, nipple discharge is normal and harmless, regardless of whether you are pregnant, breastfeeding, or neither.

Discharge from the nipple is a natural part of breast function during pregnancy or while breastfeeding. Milky discharge, also known as galactorrhea, from the nipple is common, even when you're not pregnant. The discharge after breastfeeding can continue for up to two years, even after you stop nursing. As expected, the amount that comes out of the nipple increases significantly during breastfeeding.

Milky discharge from both breasts that is non-spontaneous and copious may occur in women who have an underactive thyroid; who have growth in their pituitary gland (located in the brain), which can cause an increase prolactin levels; or as a side effect of certain medications. It is important to be evaluated by your healthcare provider to get a clearer picture of the possible causes.

Montgomery Glands and Nipple Discharge

Montgomery glands or tubercles are oil (sebaceous) glands and milk glands found on the nipple and areola. They are the bumps on the nipple that become more prominent during pregnancy. They secrete an oily substance that lubricates the skin around the nipple. They can sometimes secrete milk. Women sometimes present with a complaint of nipple discharge, but a physical examination usually demonstrates that this is normal secretion from the Montgomery glands and requires no further treatment.

The medical workup for nipple discharge starts with a physical examination. Typically, a mammogram and/or ultrasound is performed, depending on the type of nipple discharge. In the case of clear or bloody nipple discharge, an ultrasound is performed to evaluate whether there is an underlying mass that is causing the discharge. If an underlying mass is not found, referral to a breast surgeon or further evaluation with a breast MRI is performed.

Breast cancer or an intraductal papilloma (considered a high-risk lesion for breast cancer) may be the cause of clear or bloody nipple discharge. Such discharge should therefore always be reported to your doctor for further evaluation.

See your doctor immediately if you have nipple discharge that is:

- Clear, red, or bloody
- Spontaneous (comes out by itself without squeezing)
- Affecting only one breast or coming out of a single duct
- Accompanied by a breast lump

Inverted Nipples

An inverted nipple is a nipple that is turned inward. Inverted nipples are typically not a medical concern unless it's a new or worsening problem, especially on one side. New or sudden nipple inversion should always be checked by your doctor, as this can be a sign of breast cancer. Many women are born with inverted nipples or nipples that pull in at times and evert (pull out) at other times. It is common for women who are breastfeeding to experience nipple inversion, and this is usually temporary.

In some situations, especially when breastfeeding from one side more than the other, only one nipple may protrude due to the stimulation that the child's suckling provides, while the other nipple remains inverted.

Women with inverted nipples who want to breastfeed are often concerned about whether they will be able to do so. Remember that the nipple and areola are soft, pliable tissue, and the baby can adapt to your nipple to breastfeed effectively. If you are concerned about breastfeeding with an inverted nipple, seek support from a lactation consultant.

When to see your doctor: If your nipples have always protruded and you notice that they are now inverted for no apparent reason, you should see your healthcare provider, as this can be a sign of breast cancer. If you are experiencing new nipple inversion, your healthcare provider will evaluate the situation with a breast examination and breast imaging with an ultrasound and mammogram as indicated.

ASYMMETRIC BREAST SIZE

Breast asymmetry or lopsidedness is when there is a difference in the form, size, or position of your breasts. It affects more than half of all women, so know that this is a common concern.

There is no known cause for differentiated breast development, but a slight difference in the size or shape of your breasts is typically not a concern, as it merely means that one breast has more glandular tissue than the other one. The tissue in your breasts changes according to your menstrual cycle, so they may feel fuller and more sensitive between ovulation and getting your period. They can get larger due to the water retention that most women experience during this time of the month, so it is not an uncommon thing for breasts to become enlarged before menstruation and shrink during or after menstruation.

Your breasts sit on muscles and bones, so differences in muscle size or bone structure could also make one breast appear different than the other. Scoliosis (the curvature of the spine) and other deformities in the chest wall are some examples of what could affect breast size. A congenital disorder (birth defect) known as Poland syndrome can also cause unevenness. It involves the underdevelopment or absence of the chest muscles, usually on one side. These conditions may affect the appearance of breast size, but they are usually due to the condition itself, and the treatment of the underlying condition may help your breasts appear more even.

> **When to see your doctor:** In some situations, asymmetric breasts may be caused by masses in the breast tissue such as noncancerous fibroadenomas or cysts. A cancerous mass can also cause unevenness. Since there is no way to know whether a mass is a cause for concern from feeling it, you must see your doctor as soon as possible after you notice a change in breast size or shape because of a mass. Asymmetric breasts can also be the result of an infrequent problem known as juvenile hypertrophy of the breast, in which one breast grows significantly larger than the other.

If you have a sudden difference in the size or shape of one or both of your breasts, you should visit your doctor for a physical examination.

SKIN PROBLEMS

Skin issues that women can have with their breasts are usually allergy-related, or inflammatory/infectious related.

Intetrigo

Inflammation of the skin secondary to friction from the skin rubbing together is called intetrigo. Women with larger breasts are more prone to intetrigo because their breasts typically fold over the skin on their lower chest/upper abdomen. This leads to skin irritation, which, with moisture, creates a perfect environment for yeast growth. Yeast infections typically show up in the cleavage area and inframammary folds (under your breasts). They are usually caused by a yeast called candida. It can lead to skin irritation, rashes, and infections.

A red, scaly rash under your breast that may itch and cause skin discoloration could be a sign that you have a yeast infection. As with most things, it is better to prevent yeast infections than to have to treat them later. You can do this by keeping the skin under your breasts clean and dry. Intentionally lifting your breasts after a shower, to keep the area dry, is a good head start. Frequent inspection of the folds in the lower breast in front of a mirror is a good practice to notice changes early.

When to see your doctor: If problems persist despite precautions to keep the area clean and dry, your doctor can prescribe anti-fungal creams for you to apply to the affected areas.

Allergic or Contact Dermatitis

You can get a rash on your breasts related to changes in your soap and other body products. The best thing to do in this situation is to avoid using whatever is causing the rash, or it may get worse.

Eczema or Atopic Dermatitis

Typically, if you have eczema on your chest or breast area, you will have it in other parts of your body as well. It is essential to keep this type of rash well moisturized.

When to see your doctor: If the eczema is severe, you can see a skin doctor, called a dermatologist, for a stronger medication.

Acne

Unfortunately, acne caused by propionibacterium is no respecter of boundaries regarding where it can attack (ugh). Acne can occur on the skin overlying your chest and breast area. Friction from clothing, excessive sweating, hormonal fluctuations, diet, stress, and the use of harsh soap or ingredients can cause/exacerbate chest acne. You can reduce acne on the chest by washing the area daily with soap and water. If you exercise, you should remove your sweaty clothes immediately after your workout, and shower. You can also use the same over-the-counter (OTC) medication used for acne elsewhere on the body such as salicylic acid or benzoyl peroxide.

> **When to see your doctor:** If the acne persists after ensuring proper hygiene of the area, you can see a dermatologist (a skin doctor) to decide what the next best course of action is. The chest area, also known as the décolleté, is a very sensitive area of the body, even more so than the face. If OTC medications are not working, avoid the usage of harsh chemicals, as this can damage the skin in this area or exacerbate the symptoms.

Stretch Marks

Stretch marks occur when there has been rapid change in the growth of a part of your body. For example, stretch marks occur during puberty in the hips, legs, and buttocks; during pregnancy in the belly, breasts, hips, and thighs; during breastfeeding around the breasts; or during rapid weight gain or weight loss. Stretch marks often become more noticeable after the area of your body reduces in size, such as after significant weight loss or after giving birth. Theoretically, stretch marks are permanent, but they do often become less noticeable over time, depending on how severe they are.

PAGET'S DISEASE (NIPPLE BREAST CANCER)

This is a rare form of breast cancer that affects the nipple and areola (skin around the nipple). It can look like a benign (noncancerous) skin problem, such as an infection, eczema, or dermatitis, which means it is often late to be diagnosed.

Other signs of Paget's disease can include bloody nipple discharge, a sudden inversion of the nipple, skin thickening, or a lump.

If you notice any of these symptoms, it is essential that you see your doctor for a full physical examination and tests.

BREAST FULLNESS

Breast fullness typically occurs during pregnancy when your milk comes in. This may make your breasts painful and swollen. Your breasts may also feel fuller before, during, or immediately following your period. There is no cause for alarm or worry if you have breast fullness during pregnancy, breastfeeding, or around your period.

When to see your doctor: You should contact your healthcare provider for an examination if you notice any of the following:

- Breast fullness and swelling while breastfeeding with body aches, redness, fever, and pain may be signs of an infection or abscess.
- Fullness or enlargement of one of your breasts with orange-reddish skin discoloration is called "peau d'orange." If you notice this, you should **seek medical help immediately**, as this may be a sign of aggressive inflammatory breast cancer.

MASTITIS (INFECTIOUS AND NONINFECTIOUS)

Mastitis is a condition that may affect pregnant or breastfeeding women. When it isn't infectious, the symptoms include redness on the breast, pain, and lumps.

It occurs when milk ducts are obstructed due to an overproduction of milk or too much time between feedings. If duct blockage occurs, the discomfort and the lump will often dissolve after breastfeeding or pumping. If it is a persistent problem, you may be overpumping.

When to see your doctor: If you have a fever with the above symptoms, or if you have any of these symptoms while *not* breastfeeding or pregnant, it is crucial to alert your doctor. A fever usually indicates that the duct blockage has been infected, and it needs to be treated immediately, usually with antibiotics. Untreated mastitis can develop into a breast abscess.

When a breast abscess occurs, the mass is usually drained to allow for proper healing.

Cancer may be masked as mastitis, which is why an evaluation by your doctor and a breast scan with an ultrasound is very important.

ACCESSORY BREAST TISSUE

Accessory breasts are also known as supernumerary breasts, polymastia, mammae, or multiple breast syndrome. This is the condition of having non-regression of mammary tissue during embryonic development. Approximately 0.2 percent to 6 percent of the population has accessory breast tissue. It may appear with or without an areola or nipples.

Accessory breast tissue is typically felt in or around one or both armpits. In fact, some women find out that a "mole" is actually a nipple when milk comes out of it during letdown when breastfeeding! For aesthetic reasons, some people choose to remove accessory breast tissue.

If you have one or more accessory breasts, you may experience pain or tenderness, or you may feel lumps, just as you would feel in your breasts. Suspicious and concerning changes should be evaluated.

When to see your doctor: You know your breasts better than anyone, so if you notice anything unusual, including lumps, bumps, discoloration, and change in size or shape, it is essential that you schedule an examination with your healthcare provider as soon as possible.

MAIN TAKEAWAYS

Most breast complaints have a noncancerous etiology ranging from pain and infection to fibrocystic changes and benign masses. Management is often conservative with reassurance, lifestyle modifications, analgesics, or antibiotics. A thorough clinical assessment and evaluation of breast complaints by a healthcare professional is important for optimal outcomes and to ensure that breast cancer is not overlooked.

CHAPTER 4

BREAST LUMPS: A MINI-GUIDE TO THE DIFFERENT TYPES OF BREAST MASSES

IT CAN BE VERY FRIGHTENING to find a lump in your breast. It is crucial to keep in mind that a breast lump is usually benign (noncancerous). However, **a lump in your breast may be a sign of cancer**, so you must speak with a medical professional for the evaluation of any swelling or lumps you notice on your breasts.

NORMAL FIBRO-GLANDULAR BREAST TISSUE

The breasts are made up of fat, glandular tissue, fibrous connective tissue, ducts, and blood vessels. The anatomy, layout, and consistency of the breasts make them naturally feel *lumpy and bumpy*. Hormonal changes can affect the density of breast tissue, which can be perceived as a lump on physical examination. This is often apparent around the menstrual cycle and in newborns (male and female) because of the estrogen hormone passed on from their mother.

A breast lump may feel solid and unmovable, or it can feel fluid-like and roll between your fingers. Breast lumps also vary in size, from smaller than a pinhead to several inches across. They are a growth of tissue that develops inside the breast. During a physical or self-examination of the breast, a lump may be palpated. Often it is unclear whether what is being felt is normal fibro-glandular tissue. There are different types of breast lumps, and each varies in the way it feels and looks. A lump may feel like a growth, a swelling, a mass, or general fullness. With a lump, you may also notice the following:

- A firm, hard spot inside your breast.
- A lump that has distinct and definite borders.
- An area of your breast that is thicker and more prominent than the surrounding breast tissue.
- One breast is noticeably larger than the other.
- Breasts have redness, pitting, or dimpling.
- Changes in the nipple, such as being pulled inward or a discharge.
- Pain or tenderness that may increase during your menstrual cycle.

DIFFERENT TYPES OF BREAST MASSES/LUMPS

Sometimes a lump in the breast is a sign of breast cancer, which is why it is crucial to seek prompt medical attention if you do notice a breast mass or lump. Fortunately, most breast lumps are the result of benign, noncancerous conditions.

Most benign breast lumps are related to your menstrual cycle and fluctuation in your hormones. Other benign breast lumps may be due to an infection, a breast injury, or plugged milk ducts.

Some of the most common causes of benign breast masses and/or lumps include the following:

- **Breast cysts:** Fluid-filled sacs within your breast. They are often tender to the touch and may come and go with your menstrual period.
- **Fibrocystic breasts:** Breast tissue that feels granular or ropy. Fibrocystic breasts include symptoms such as being tender to the touch and a thickening of tissue. These changes are often related to a fluctuation in hormones and may increase in middle age but disappear during menopause.
- **Lipoma:** Fat-containing breast mass that is typically benign.
- **Fat necrosis:** Occurs when there is an injury to the fatty breast tissue, resulting in firm, round lumps.

- **Mastitis:** Inflammation from breast tissue, which can be infectious or noninfectious. **Note**: Inflammatory breast cancer, which is an aggressive form of breast cancer, can look like mastitis. Therefore, follow-up when being treated for mastitis is important, especially if the symptoms are getting worse or there is no improvement with treatment.
- *Infectious mastitis* includes an infection and generally occurs in women who are breastfeeding due to a combination of pooled breast milk and bacteria from an infant's mouth.
- *Granulomatous mastitis* is a rare benign inflammatory condition. The typical presentation is like that of infectious mastitis, where there is a complaint of skin redness, a lump, and sometimes discharge. Although a self-limiting and benign condition, it can progress to cause skin ulcerations, abscesses, and fistula formation. After four to six weeks of no improvement from a presumed infection, a biopsy is performed to exclude cancer or an inadequately treated infection.
- **Cellular Fibroepithelial Lesions (CFEL)**
- *Fibroadenoma*: The most common benign and noncancerous tumor of the breast. It occurs usually in young women aged fifteen to thirty-five but can occur at any age. It typically does not turn into cancer. It is usually managed conservatively with clinical and imaging follow-up. However, complex fibroadenomas and any fibroadenoma that is rapidly growing or causing symptoms are usually surgically removed.
- *Phyllodes*: A rare tumor that makes up less than 1 percent of all breast tumors. It is formed from the connective tissues of the breast. Seventy-five percent of phyllodes are benign and about 15 percent are malignant (cancerous). It is not the same cancer as breast cancer. A malignant phyllodes tumor spreads through the blood, and a chest imaging study is often obtained to look for lung metastasis. All phyllodes tumors are surgically removed.

FREQUENTLY ASKED QUESTIONS ABOUT BENIGN AND MALIGNANT LUMPS

Can You Tell if a Lump Is Cancerous or Malignant When You Touch It?

A painless and fixed lump in the breast should not be brushed off, as it may be a malignant tumor. In general, a lump that is fluid-filled and mobile, such as a simple cyst, is less likely to be cancerous, while a lump that is hard and fixed may be a sign of cancer. These typical observations are not set in stone; some cancerous lumps may be mobile, and some benign lumps may be fixed. Since humans don't have touch or X-ray vision capabilities to determine if a palpable lump is malignant or benign, all lumps should be evaluated by your healthcare provider and medical imaging should be obtained to better characterize a lump as benign or suspicious for malignancy.

Are Cancerous Lumps Painful?

Pain may or may not be associated with breast cancer. The absence or presence of pain should not be used as a form of prediction or diagnosis of what a lump could be. It still needs to be evaluated by a healthcare professional for determination of next steps, which is usually a diagnostic image evaluation.

Do Benign Lumps Require Testing?

Not all lumps are cancerous. However, I do believe that all lumps require evaluation by a healthcare professional and imaging evaluation. A medical expert who understands evidence-based breast care protocols will typically order imaging to rule out malignancy. If diagnostic imaging determines a lump is suspicious, tissue sampling (typically with a needle biopsy) is performed for definitive diagnosis.

Lumps during Pregnancy and Lactation and Other Issues

During pregnancy, the milk ducts prepare for breastfeeding. Thus, the breasts become heavier and larger in size, and they can also become more sensitive and tender during pregnancy and lactation. Below you will read about some of the most common changes that can occur in the breasts during pregnancy and breastfeeding.

Normal Breast Tissue and Clogged Ducts

The most common cause of breast lumps during pregnancy is the swelling of the milk-producing glands. The swelling may cause your breasts to feel more lumpy than usual.

While clogged ducts are typically experienced after childbirth, during lactation or weaning, women who start producing milk during pregnancy can also experience clogged ducts. This can be painful; it can feel like a hard lump and may develop into a breast infection (mastitis). Continuing to breastfeed is typically the only intervention needed.

Fibroadenoma

A breast lump that can occur and increase in size during pregnancy or while breastfeeding is a fibroadenoma. These masses are smooth, firm, rubbery, and mobile. It is a common type of breast lump, and they do not significantly increase your risk of breast cancer. Unless a fibroadenoma is causing problems, your doctor will usually recommend that it be left alone and managed with observation.

NONINFECTIOUS AND INFECTIOUS MASTITIS AND ABSCESSES

When your breasts begin to produce milk, and the milk is not removed from the breast by your baby drinking it or by pumping, it can cause clogged ducts. A clogged duct feels like a hard, painful lump, and it might cause redness or warmth on the skin above it. If you detect a clogged duct early on, you can clear the duct simply by breastfeeding your baby or pumping your milk. Some women also find relief by massaging the area or using hot compresses.

However, if the clogged duct is not cleared promptly, mastitis, which is an infection of the breast tissue, can develop. This can be very painful, and most women need to take antibiotics to clear it up. One may notice a warmth and redness of the skin overlying the breast. If you have mastitis, you should not stop breastfeeding or pumping, as it can make the problem worse.

If mastitis is not cleared up, an abscess can develop, and you may need to be aspirated or surgically drained. A fever, chills, nausea, and vomiting are signs of a systemic infection and require prompt notification of your healthcare provider.

Nipple Discharge

As your breasts prepare for lactation during pregnancy, some women notice a clear, yellowish, or white discharge from their nipples, especially toward the end of the third trimester. This is normal and should not be cause for concern. If you notice a bloody tinge, however, you should call your doctor immediately.

Galactocele

A mass that can form from duct obstruction is called a galactocele or lactocele, which is a milk cyst. It is the most common mass detected during the period of lactation, and it can also occur during weaning. Diagnosis is made with imaging using a mammogram and ultrasound. In most cases, these masses resolve on their own.

Lactating Adenoma

This is a rare and benign breast tumor that occurs late in pregnancy or during the early postpartum period. It usually appears due to rising estrogen levels and can grow quickly. It is often self-limited and typically resolves after delivery or the cessation of breastfeeding. If it is large or has a complex appearance, tissue sampling may be required to attain a definitive diagnosis.

PREGNANCY ASSOCIATED BREAST CANCER (PABC)

Pregnancy associated breast cancer is rare (1 in 3,000 women); it may occur in a woman during pregnancy, up to twelve months after giving birth, or at any time during lactation. It is the most common malignancy in pregnant women. Due to the hormonal and physical changes that occur in a woman's breasts during pregnancy and lactation, PABC is usually detected at an advanced stage with a high mortality rate. PABC is considered aggressive due to detection in younger patients with larger-size tumors, lymph node involvement at diagnosis, aggressive immunochemistry with negative estrogen and progesterone receptors, and overexpression of human epidermal growth factor (HER-2). Due to decreased mammographic sensitivity and non-ionization radiation, an ultrasound is the first-line imaging modality of choice in a pregnant or breastfeeding patient. Although most masses during pregnancy and lactation are benign, it is of utmost importance to report new or growing masses during pregnancy or lactation promptly to a healthcare provider.

BREAST LUMPS IN MEN

Male breasts, like female breasts, are made up of fat and fibrous tissue and have an interconnecting system of breast ducts. Small lymph nodes are occasionally present in male breasts and are usually in the outer portion of the breast, near the underarm.

One of the most common causes for an increase in breast tissue in males is a noncancerous disorder known as gynecomastia. It usually appears as a lump or swelling in one or both breasts; it is usually centrally located behind the nipple and may be tender to the touch.

Breast cancer is possible in males, although uncommon (less than 1 percent of males). It occurs most often in males between the ages of sixty and seventy but may occur at any age. Usually, breast cancer in men is presented with a hard, painless lump that is typically under the nipple. Although it is rare, fibroadenomas may also occur in male breasts as fibrous tumors, inflammatory masses, or enlarged lymph nodes.

MAIN TAKEAWAYS

It is important to remember that most breast lumps are noncancerous.

However, if you discover a new lump, an area of your breast that is significantly different from the rest, a lump that does not go away, grows larger, or changes, and/or your breast is bruised for no apparent reason, it is important to visit your doctor as soon as possible.

It is extremely important that you talk with your medical provider to learn how to do a self-examination and that you have mammograms and physical examinations as ordered by your doctor.

SECTION 3

BREAST CANCER: FACTS, DIAGNOSIS, TREATMENT, AND SURVIVORSHIP.

The epidemiology of breast cancers, looking at the incidence, prevalence, and survival rate for symptomatic and screen-detected breast cancers. Diagnosis, treatment, and beyond.

CHAPTER 5

BREAST CANCER FACTS

KNOWING THE FACTS ABOUT BREAST CANCER can help you understand your risks so you can make sure you get the preventive care you need to stay healthy. Here's what you need to know.

WHAT IS BREAST CANCER?

Breast cancer is a disease that causes changes in the growth and development of cells within the breast tissue. Cancer cells in the breast form tumors, which appear as lumps inside the breast. Breast cancer can occur in the milk glands (or lobules), the milk ducts, or the tissue itself. Breast cancer can form in the ducts in what is known as an *in situ*—meaning non-invasive, but with the potential to become invasive with the ability to metastasize. Non-invasive forms of breast cancer indicate an increased risk for the development of an invasive malignancy if left untreated. Breast cancers can also be invasive, meaning they can break through the walls of the ducts or glands and can spread to the surrounding breast tissue and elsewhere in the body.

HOW COMMON IS BREAST CANCER AROUND THE WORLD?

Worldwide, breast cancer is the most common type of cancer in women. More than half a million women die of breast cancer each year, and the number of breast cancer cases is about equal in both developed and less-developed countries, with more deaths occurring in less-developed countries. According to the World Health Organization (WHO), 2.3 million women were diagnosed with breast cancer in 2020, with

685,000 deaths globally. By the end of 2020, 7.8 million with a diagnosis of breast cancer in the past five years were alive. There are more lost disability-adjusted life years (DALYs) by women to breast cancer globally than any other type of cancer. The greatest risk factors for breast cancer are being a woman and increasing age.

Prevalence rates vary significantly among different areas of the world; however, even in areas where breast cancer rates have traditionally been low, such as East Africa, the incidence of breast cancer has been steadily increasing. Survival rates also vary, ranging from about 80 percent in Japan, Sweden, and the United States to less than 40 percent in low-income countries.

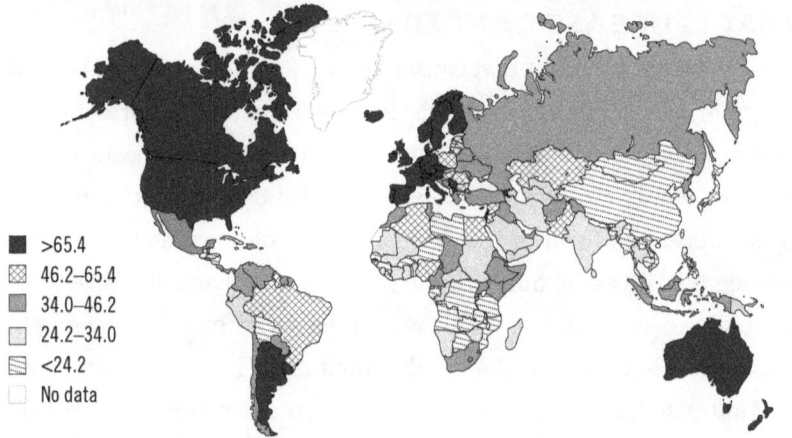

Estimated age-standardized rates of incident cases, breast cancer, worldwide in 2012

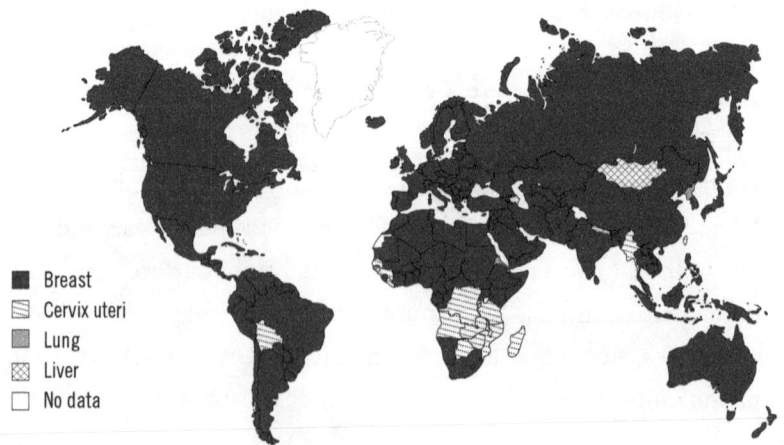

Top cancer per country, estimated number of new cases, females, all ages, in 2020

The map on the previous page illustrates that there are fewer incidences of breast cancer in African populations than in North America and Australia. It is important to note that while there may be fewer cases due to lifestyle factors, women in Africa may also be less commonly diagnosed, even if they do develop breast cancer, due to low awareness and weaker healthcare systems.

Estimated age-standardized rates of deaths, breast cancer, worldwide in 2012

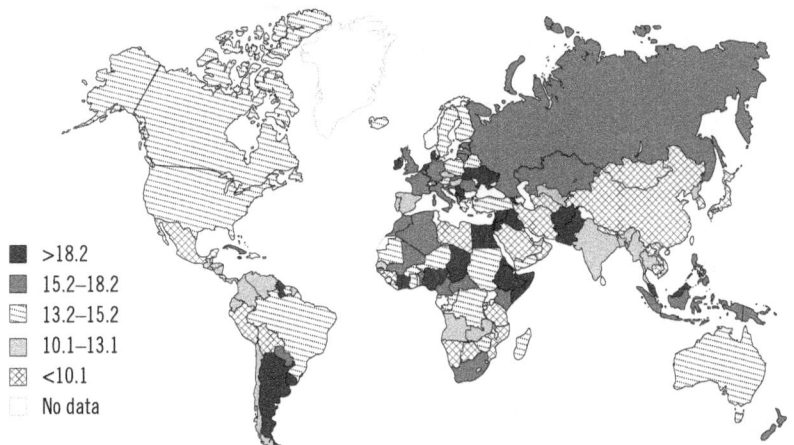

Top cancer per country, estimated number of new cases, females, all ages, in 2020

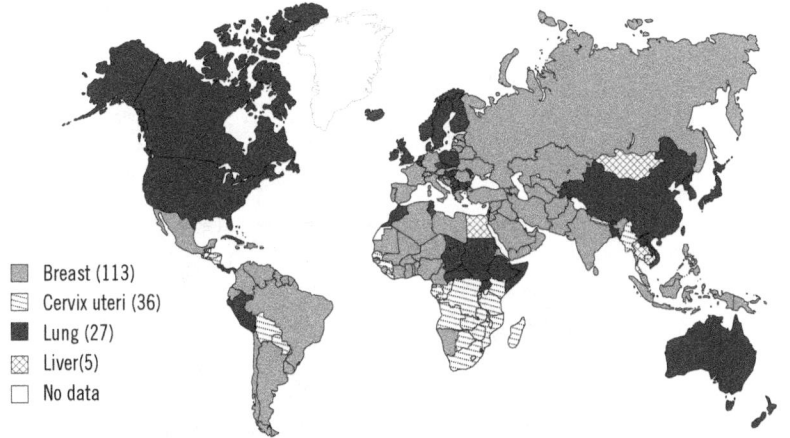

Even though a person from Africa is less likely to develop breast cancer than people in regions with higher rates like the United States and Australia, she is more likely to die of breast cancer. This also has to do with low awareness and poor access to healthcare.

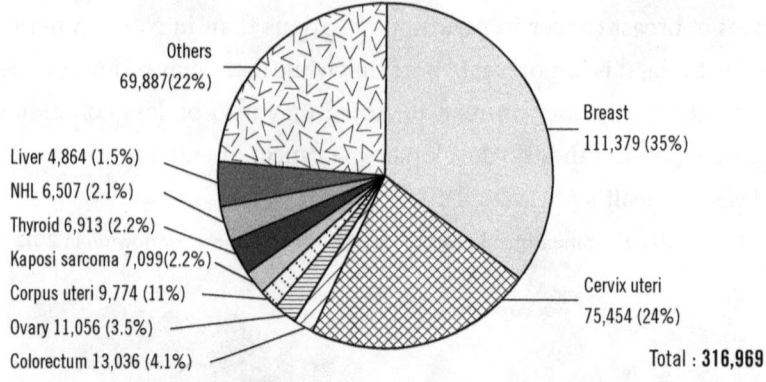

In the pie chart above, the World Health Organization demonstrates that breast cancer is the most common type of cancer in Africa; 35 percent of all diagnosed cancer cases are breast cancer.

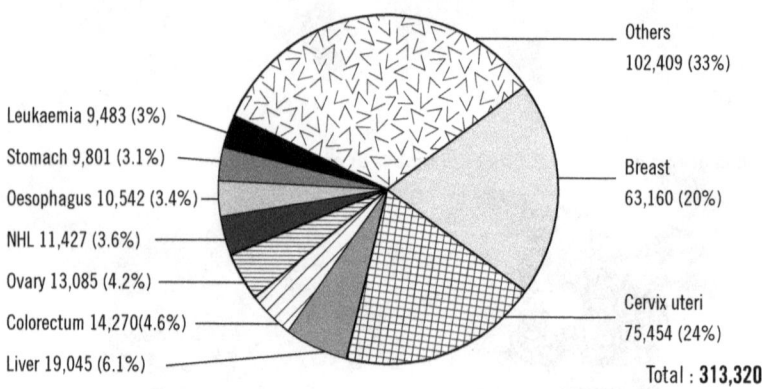

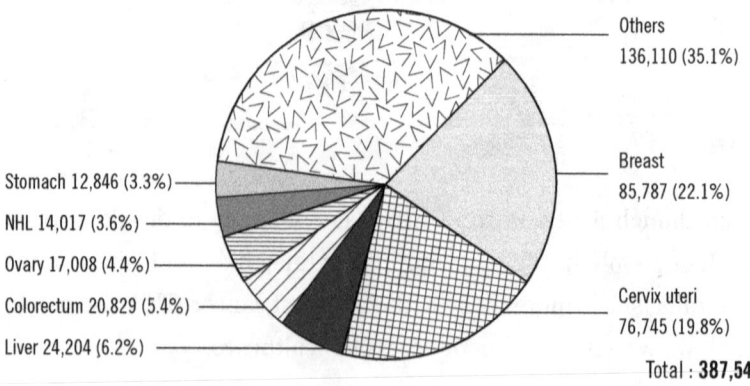

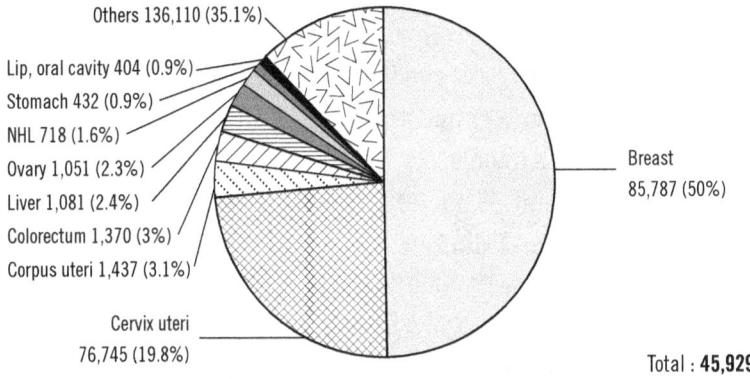

Estimated number of prevalence cases (1-year), Nigeria (top 10 cancer sites) in 2012

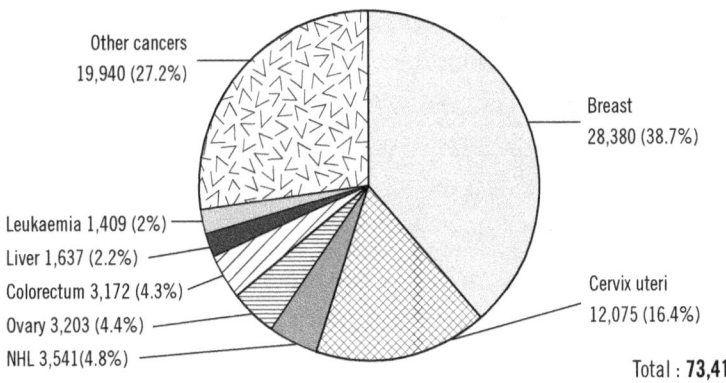

Estimated number of new cases in 2020, Nigeria, females, all ages

About 20 percent of deaths in Africa are linked to breast cancer.

Nigeria has one of the highest prevalence of breast cancer; 50 percent of total diagnosed cancers in Nigeria are due to breast cancer.

HOW COMMON IS BREAST CANCER IN AFRICA?

Cancer is an emerging health problem in Africa. In 2012, there were over 847,000 diagnosed cancer cases and 591,000 cancer deaths. These numbers are expected to double in the next twenty years based on population growth and the increase in life expectancy.

Other reasons we expect to see an increase in the incidence of cancer is an increase in the popularity of the Western lifestyle, which includes smoking, sedentary lifestyles, and obesity.

Another reason for the predicted rise in cancer is the high rate of cancer-causing infectious organisms. For example, the Human Papillomavirus (HPV) causes cervical cancer; Hepatitis B and Hepatitis C both cause liver cancer; and the Human Immunodeficiency Virus (HIV) causes Kaposi sarcoma.

Due to the implementation of screening programs and better treatment regimens, cancer death rates are on the decline in Western countries. However, the trend is the opposite in low- and middle-income countries. In my research of the scientific data, this trend is projected to increase exponentially. For instance, of the 14.1 million incident cases and 8.2 million deaths that occurred worldwide in 2012 due to cancer, 60 percent of the new cases and 72 percent of the deaths occurred in low- and middle-income countries.

So, although the overall global data for cancer in the world is higher in Western countries, the number of deaths from cancer is higher in less developed countries. This is mainly due to a lack of early detection and access to treatment facilities.

Nigeria is the most populous country in Africa. Breast cancer is the most common malignancy in Nigeria, surpassing prostate and cervical cancer (in that order). Scientific and research data suggest that breast cancer develops at a younger age in patients of African descent as compared to Caucasians. The peak incidence of breast cancer in a Nigerian woman has been reported to be under the age of fifty, which is about a decade earlier than in Caucasians. The five-year breast cancer survival rate in Nigeria is reported to be between 10 percent and 35 percent, compared with between 70 percent and 90 percent in Western Europe and North America. The primary factor associated with this disparity in survival is the delay in detection, diagnosis, and treatment of breast cancer due to poor awareness, which limits treatment options.

MAIN TAKEAWAYS

Early detection of breast cancer requires early diagnosis in symptomatic women and regular screening in asymptomatic women. Multiple published studies have shown the benefit of early detection in the treatment and survival outcomes of breast cancer.

The American Cancer Society considers mammography to be an effective method of early detection, since it can identify cancer several years before physical symptoms develop. The Society of Breast Imaging recommends annual breast cancer screening in women who are forty years of age or older.

Therefore, the development of initiatives that give access to quality and affordable breast cancer screening to all women regardless of geographic location is essential.

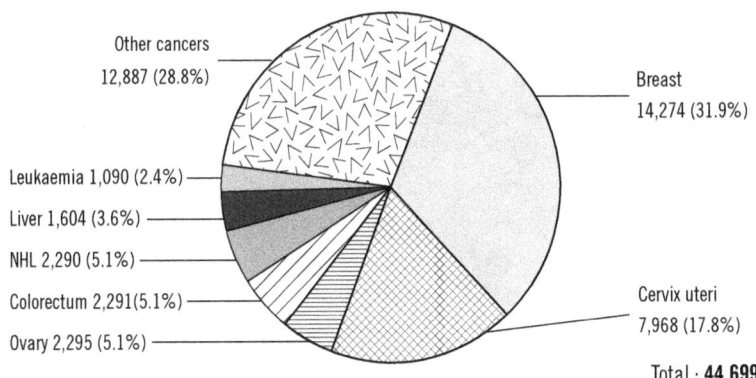

Estimated number of deaths in 2020, Nigeria, females, all ages

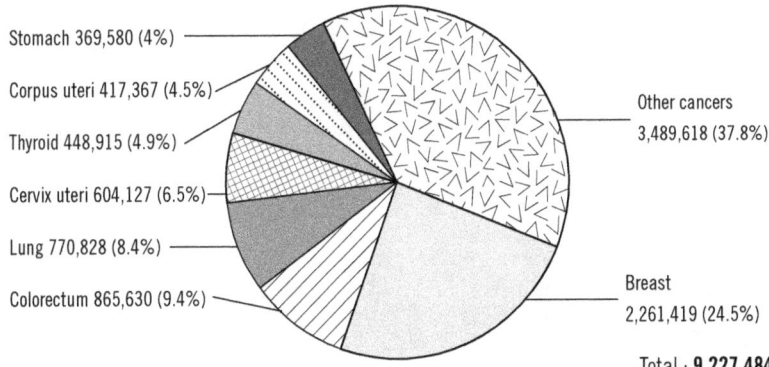

Estimated number of new cases in 2020, world, females, all ages

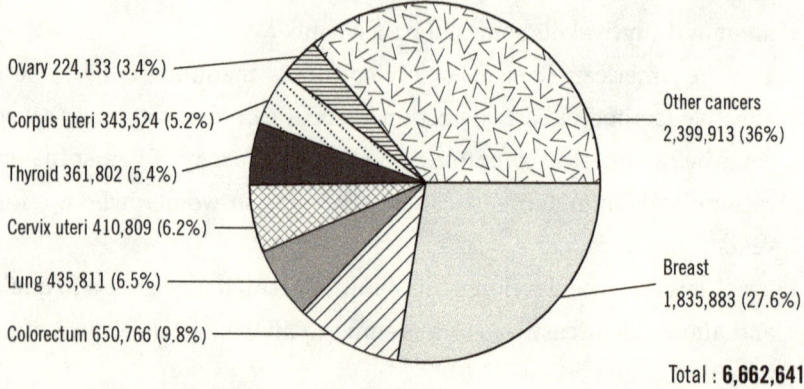

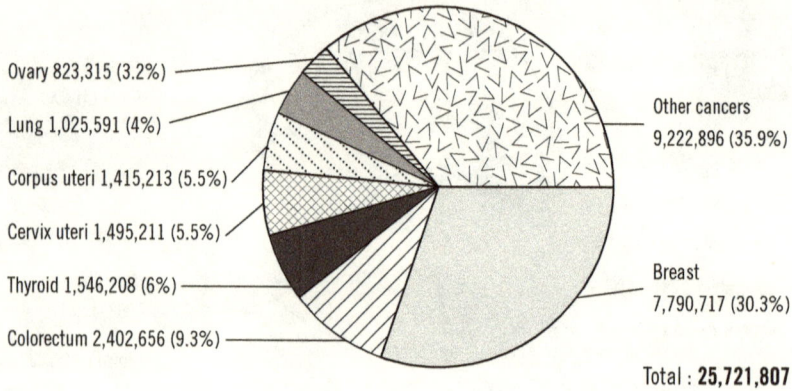

CHAPTER 6
FEAR AND BREAST CANCER: YOU'RE NOT ALONE

FEAR OF CANCER DIAGNOSIS

If you're a woman who fears breast cancer, please know that it is understandable, and you are not alone. A cancer diagnosis is serious and never a walk in the park at any stage. However, the fear of a cancer diagnosis can be disabling. For example, in some settings, the thought alone is strong enough to trigger panic, anxiety, and depression, even in the absence of an actual diagnosis. This is called *carcinophobia*, a debilitating fear and anxiety of getting cancer. It's typically seen in people who have had cancer or have witnessed it in another person, usually a close relative or friend. Some people fear the disease enough to only refer to it as the "C-word," not daring to even utter the name out loud. The stigma and fatalistic health beliefs surrounding cancer fuel myths and misinformation, which unfortunately end up being counterproductive for early detection of cancer.

Horror stories, radical therapies, and a deep-rooted stigma associated with the disease being "terminal" contribute to the widespread fear. Fear of breast cancer is legitimate, says cancer survivor Peggy Orenstein. But she also notes that women's responses to, and emotions surrounding, the fear "can be manipulated, packaged, marketed, and sold, sometimes by the very forces that claim to support us."

What Can Help

"Most people think their risk of getting breast cancer for the first time is higher than it really is," says BreastCancer.org. Get the truth by talking to your doctor, or a specialized healthcare professional who can assess your risk based on your personal risk factors. You may find your risk is much lower than you feared. Dispelling myths that fuel the cancer stigma is crucial.

Secondly, be kind to yourself despite feeling this way. Take solace in knowing there are millions of women who share similar fears about breast cancer as you do. Knowing you're not alone should help ease some of the anxiety from the get-go. Figuring out what scares you the most, and then taking action to alleviate those worries, can help ease it even more.

FEAR OF THE MAMMOGRAM

Turning forty can be a big deal for many women for a lot of reasons. As they say, "Life begins at forty"—and it is also the beginning of your recommended annual screening mammogram. Fear of this examination and what to expect, especially for the first one, can cause a delay in its initiation. There's no shortage of dreadful tales you may have heard, such as that the test is painful, embarrassing, and mushes your breast like a pancake.

What Can Help

Your breasts won't be totally flattened like a pancake, as you might imagine. They will, however, be positioned between two plates: an immobile bottom plate and adjustable top one, both of which are attached to a large mammogram machine. You'll stand near the machine in various positions while the technician takes a few X-rays of each breast. While the examination is not exactly pleasant, it is not as excruciatingly painful as depicted. It's also typically over rather quickly, with each image only taking a few seconds to capture.

Tip

Always feel free to communicate with the technician/radiographer who acquires your images about any discomfort you may have, as well as about what you need to help relieve your anxiety (for example, knowing when you can expect the results, etc.).

MAIN TAKEAWAYS

The risk for developing breast cancer increases as you age. Starting an annual mammogram habit at age forty can get you in the regular groove of making the most of early detection methods. The earlier the cancer is detected, the better. Don't let the fear of a breast cancer diagnosis stop you from being proactive.

CHAPTER 7

BREAST CANCER STIGMA AND MYTHS

Because people feel stigmatized, they don't want to talk about it, and in not talking about it, a lot of myths and misconceptions are increased and allowed to spread.
—*Claire Neal*, Principal Investigator, "Cancer Stigma and Silence around the World: A LiveStrong Foundation Report"

"STIGMA" CAN BE DEFINED AS A KIND of mark of shame or disgrace. E. Goffman defined "stigma" as a reduction of a person to less than whole, as tainted and discounted. Stigma can often be firmly attached to several health conditions such as alcoholism, drug abuse, mental health, and a variety of other diseases—like breast cancer.

Breast cancer comes with numerous stigmas in tow, often bringing shame and disgrace to the women who suffer from the disease. As if they had a choice. As if being diagnosed with breast cancer was somehow their doing.

SURVIVOR INSIGHT: PJ HAMEL

Writer and fourteen-year breast cancer survivor PJ Hamel says that the diagnosis of cancer changes your life forever. "One moment, you're a face in the crowd, part of the vast majority of people who go through life assuming good health. And then, after a few simple words from your doctor, that world is lost to you forever."

She says the new, changing world of cancer often comes with:

- Averted gazes from everyone you encounter, especially if you have the physical symptoms of someone going through chemotherapy such as hair loss.
- Uncomfortable small talk from acquaintances, friends, and family.
- Family members who treat you differently, no longer joking or even nagging like they used to.
- Friends who may become closer, stick around for a spell, then disappear until you recover or fade away forever.

Hamel adds that the "cancer survivor" label marks you as a person who has been there, and someone who always has the chance of going back. She even asked her oncologist when she could officially say she's cured of cancer. He told her, "When you die of something else." Yikes!

IMPACT ON DEVELOPING NATIONS

The stigma and myths associated with breast cancer are especially commonplace in developing nations, as noted by the *New York Times* and the Union for International Cancer Control (UICC). While about 20 percent of breast cancer patients die from the disease in the United States, that rate is as high as 40 percent to 60 percent in poorer countries. The higher death rates can be attributed to several factors such as poverty, erroneous information, lack of awareness—and the stigma associated with the disease. All these factors work together to cause some women to avoid seeking help until it's too late.

SURVIVOR INSIGHT: MARY NAMATA

A *New York Times* article examining the state of breast cancer in Uganda told the story of Mary Namata, age forty-eight, who lives in Budd, a village outside Kamala, Uganda. In Budd, there's no word for "cancer" in the native language. Mary was first evaluated by a visiting team of American doctors. By this time, she already had multiple breast masses pulling her skin so tight that it appeared as if they might burst through the skin.

Four years prior, she had sought help from a local doctor when she first noticed a single lump in her right breast. The doctor informed her that the breast would probably have to be removed. Her elderly mother angrily protested that no woman should have her breast cut off.

In Africa, a mastectomy (which is a surgical procedure to remove all or part of a breast to treat breast cancer or prevent it in women with high lifetime risk) is a more common procedure than breast conservation with lumpectomy (which is the partial removal of breast tissue). This is because the technology and resources needed to ensure negative margins (i.e., all the cancer cells are removed) and adequate treatment for breast conservation is very limited or lacking.

Mary's Journey with Breast Cancer Treatments

Mary was ready to have a mastectomy, but friends and relatives talked her out of it by saying it would cause the cancer to spread and kill her. So, she decided to try herbal treatments instead. Herbal treatments were popular and widely available in her village, and they were hawked for treating everything from syphilis to diabetes, with cancer in between.

Mary's daughter took out a loan to secure these herbal treatments, but her mother's tumors just kept growing. They brought pain so severe she could no longer sleep at night.

Her intense pain finally prompted her to visit a breast clinic in Mulago, which requires two buses and two scooter taxi rides to get to. This was where she encountered the visiting American team of doctors, who gave her a checkup with available resources. They suggested using chemotherapy to shrink the tumors and make it easier to perform a mastectomy. She eventually began treatment, and the tumors started to shrink in size.

Even after the initial doubt about the effectiveness of technological-based treatments, Mary was able to access the care she needed to manage her breast cancer.

SURVIVOR INSIGHT: OYINDA BALOGUN

Oyinda, aged fifty-six, lives in an uncompleted building with her young children and husband on the outskirts of Lagos, Nigeria. She was a petty trader doing all she could to make ends meet for her family when she discovered a lump in her breast when taking a shower. She told her family and friends, and they encouraged her to take herbal supplements and increase her intake of fruits and vegetables. Several months went by and the lump kept growing. During a free mammogram screening event at church, she summoned the courage to ask one of the coordinators if she could be a beneficiary. She got a mammogram, which described a mass that was three centimeters. An ultrasound confirmed a mass, and biopsy was suggested. She did not have the financial means to obtain the procedure. Once again, her family and friends encouraged herbal supplements and an uptake of fruits and vegetables. The mass continued to grow. It was becoming painful.

Oyinda's Journey with Breast Cancer Treatment

Oyinda summoned the courage to approach one of the medical outreach coordinators at church and her pastor. They encouraged her to seek medical intervention promptly, as her complaints were worrisome and indicative of breast cancer. It had been almost a year since she first discovered the lump in her breast, and her symptoms had advanced considerably. A repeat ultrasound now showed multiple masses and enlarged lymph nodes in her armpit. A biopsy confirmed a triple positive cancer, which is a type of breast cancer that tests positive for three specific receptors: estrogen receptors (ER+), progesterone receptors (PR+), and human epidermal growth factor receptor 2 (HER2+). This type of cancer can respond well to targeted therapies that block these receptors, offering more treatment options compared to cancers that aren't positive for these receptors—but it would cost an astronomical amount of money to treat, money she and her family did not have. She was devastated.

After crowdfunding from friends, family, and social-media well-wishers, she was only able to raise a minuscule amount of money.

Time was ticking, and there was no place for her to turn. Fortunately, one of the medical outreach coordinators at her church was able to locate a trial for patients with HER2+ cancers. She qualified for the program and was able to receive treatment. She completed therapy within six months, including having a mastectomy.

Today, her cancer is in remission. She welcomed a new grandchild and lived to celebrate another birthday. She now supports women in her community who are facing a new diagnosis of breast cancer, and she uses her story to encourage other women through their treatment journey.

THE SOCIAL CHALLENGES OF BREAST CANCER TREATMENT IN DEVELOPING COUNTRIES

Mary's and Oyinda's stories are inspiring, but they are the exception. Most women in low-income countries don't have successful outcomes when it comes to breast cancer: their disease is often caught late; they don't have any avenues for diagnosis and treatment (nor the means to afford such treatment); and they are often given incorrect advice thanks to stigma, poor awareness, and the very real social challenges of breast cancer in developing countries.

The world of breast cancer in developing countries often comes with:

- Women being left by their husbands or boyfriends.
- Women being fired from work for taking time off for treatment.
- Families keeping cancer a secret, fearing no one will marry their daughters or interact with the family if the disease is found out.
- Darkened skin from chemotherapy treatments, which can peg the women as having AIDS because darkened skin is one of the side effects of HIV treatment.
- Women with one breast after a mastectomy being shunned, either for being cursed by a witch or for being witches themselves.

WHY THE STIGMA?

The cancer stigma is rampant across the world, according to a LiveStrong report that interviewed more than 4,500 cancer survivors, healthcare providers, community members, and organizational leaders across ten countries. The report uncovered a universal "stigma index" that includes views like the following:

- Support and treatment are pointless for someone with cancer.
- I would not be comfortable being friends with someone who has cancer.
- I would feel alone and isolated if I had to undergo cancer treatment.
- I'd consider leaving my spouse if he or she had cancer.
- People can only blame themselves for getting cancer.
- Cancer is a spiritual disease, either punishment or attack from one's enemies.

Several factors fuel the cancer stigma, says Claire Neal, a team member of the LiveStrong anti-stigma campaign. The main factor is the lack of understanding of how and why cancer develops. Its development has been blamed on everything from witchcraft to stress, from a judgment from God to unhealthy habits and poor hygiene. Herein lie the seeds for blaming people for bringing the disease on themselves.

Fears that cancer is contagious fuel the stigma further. Cancer survivors may be shunned by neighbors, friends, and the community. Families can break apart, and lifelong relationships can be ruined.

The numerous ways in which cancer and its treatment can affect a person externally and internally are another cause for stigmatization. Cancer can affect:

- How a person looks.
- How a person feels.
- Their sexuality.
- Their ability to have children.
- Their behavior and relationships with family and friends.

"There are so many ways that cancer and its treatment can impact a person's life," Neal points out, "and there has been this silence around it."

Allowing stigmas surrounding cancer to go unchecked marginalizes health-seeking behaviors, propagates myths and beliefs that may prompt a woman to stop treatment, and curtails even the consideration of seeking medical advice when there is a concern.

BUSTING NINE COMMON BREAST CANCER MYTHS

Myths surrounding breast cancer add another layer of fuel to the stigma fire. Some of the most common myths outlined by the National Cancer Institute and the National Breast Cancer Coalition include the following.

Myth #9: A lump in your breast automatically means you have breast cancer.

Fact: Most breast lumps turn out *not* to be cancer, but no lump should be ignored. Getting it checked out with a clinical breast exam is the wisest move to relieve your fears—and dispel the myth.

Myth #8: Men never get breast cancer.

Fact: Men *can* get breast cancer. Estimates say about 1 percent of diagnosed breast cancers are in men, resulting in about 410 deaths each year. Men can perform the same type of self-exams women do, bringing any issues or concerns to their doctors.

Myth #7: Radiation from mammograms is very dangerous.

Fact: Even though mammograms involve the use of X-rays, the radiation levels are extremely low. The benefits of early detection outweigh the risk of radiation exposure. In fact, there is a similar amount of radiation, if not more, when you travel by air from Lagos to New York.

To help put the radiation dose concern in perspective, according to the American Cancer Society, people in the United States are normally exposed to an average of about 3 **millisieverts** (mSv) of radiation each year just from their natural surroundings. This is called *background radiation*. The dose of radiation used for a screening mammogram of both breasts is about the same amount of radiation a woman would get from her natural surroundings in just over seven weeks. On average, the total dose for a typical mammogram with two views of each breast is about 0.4 mSv. Put another way, you would be exposed to **about 0.035 mSv (3.5 mrem)** of cosmic radiation if you were to fly within the United States from the east to west coast.

This risk is also limited by choosing a reputable facility that follows industry standards and requirements of certifying bodies like the Mammography Quality Standards Acts (MQSA) for the maintenance and operation of mammography equipment.

Myth #6: Mammograms can cause cancer to spread.
Fact: The compression used to perform a mammogram is just enough to hold the breast still so that the images obtained are of diagnostic quality.

Myth #5: Mammograms prevent breast cancer.
Fact: Although mammograms cannot prevent cancer, they help detect it so you can act at the earliest stages.

Myth #4: You're highly likely to develop breast cancer if your family has a history of it.
Fact: Although a family history of breast cancer does put women at greater risk, only about 10 percent of people diagnosed with breast cancer have a family history of it.

Myth #3: Breast cancer is contagious.
Fact: You cannot "catch" cancer from someone else or transmit it if you have it. Breast cancer comes from the uncontrolled growth of mutant

cells that can spread to other tissues within the breast and body. You cannot get it from your neighbor.

Myth #2: Removing the entire breast with a mastectomy increases chances of survival better than just removing the cancer and undergoing radiation treatments.

Fact: Scientific research studies have shown that mastectomies are typically not more effective than lumpectomy with radiation therapy for breast cancer treatment. Each cancer is different; each patient is different. A multidisciplinary breast oncology team helps tailor cancer therapy in a manner that is appropriate for each patient using evidence-based guidelines.

Myth #1: Cancer is a death sentence.

Cancer is not an automatic death sentence.

Breast cancer survivor Peggy Orenstein points out, "Breast cancer in your breast doesn't kill you; the disease becomes deadly when it metastasizes, spreading to other organs or the bones." She additionally notes that breast cancer death rates have dropped about 25 percent since 1990.

Treatments have come a long way, squashing the myth that nothing can be done about cancer. Living a healthy life and practicing prevention measures may also reduce the risk.

Cancer doesn't specifically target the elderly, wealthy, or people in developed countries. It can affect people of all ages, economic statuses, and regions. Living in a developed country, however, means you're likely to have more advanced treatment options available.

FEAR OF LOSING A BREAST

Losing a breast can make women fear that they'll lose their femininity, that their spouses or lovers will no longer find them attractive, or that they'll no longer be a "whole woman." Again, none of these fears need to be true.

What Can Help

A mastectomy is by no means the only treatment option in every situation, nor is it even always the recommended one. Depending on the type of cancer and various other factors, treatment options can range from chemotherapy to hormone therapy. A mastectomy is not always a recommended preventative option, either.

True, Angelina Jolie made headlines with her risk-reducing double mastectomy, but such a move may not be indicated for everyone.

Treatment options should be tailored to the patient. Reconstructive surgery is just one of the options that can be taken, following a mastectomy. Prosthetic bras with built-in padding are also widely available. Women can also find specialized bathing suits, lingerie, loungewear, and even molded breast inserts designed to fit inside a bra cup. Other women with mastectomies have taken an artistic approach, adorning their chests with elaborate tattoos.

ARMING YOURSELF WITH THE FACTS: BREAKING THE VICIOUS CYCLE OF MISINFORMATION

The fear of the unknown is universal, and it stems from several causes. In the most basic sense, we often fear the unknown because, well, we don't know what's waiting for us. It could be something terrible. It could be something that gets us into trouble. It could be something that makes us lose what we already have.

Worse yet, if we don't know what's out there waiting for us, there is no way we can control it. That may be what scares us the most: we are afraid of having absolutely no control, no way to guide or manipulate a situation to the outcome we want.

In all honesty, we don't have control over anything. Sure, we can take certain actions in the hopes of creating specific outcomes, but we never truly know what's going to happen tomorrow, after lunch, or even two minutes down the line. You have two ways to handle fear of the unknown. One is to become paralyzed and wallow in fear, and the other is to be courageous by acting.

Is There a Way to Ease Fears?

As always, talking to others about your fears and concerns goes a long way. Sharing your fears with others can help you realize that you are not alone. Getting fear out of your head and into the open deflates its power and hold. Instead of letting your fears fester in your brain, where your imagination can make them seem infinitely worse, put your fears on the table and look them square in the eye. Courage is action despite fear.

Another aspect to look at is where you are now considering some of the things you were afraid of in the past. Looking back, you've likely learned that moving forward despite your fears puts you in a new, albeit unknown, place, and that the new place typically ends up being an upgrade. Being paralyzed in fear is not fun—shifting your state out of fear to a state of possibilities, hope, and courage is a win-win.

Arming yourself with information about the unknown is another wise move, mainly because it takes away the mystery and uncertainty associated with fear. For instance, if your fear of breast cancer stems from not knowing much about the disease, arm yourself with power by reading up on it, like you're doing now. Talk to your doctor about it. Speak with people who have been through it. Seek answers for whatever questions or uncertainties you may have.

While you still won't have control over what happens, you'll at least have solid knowledge and a better sense of what's making you so afraid. This, in turn, will give you a better sense of confidence.

MAIN TAKEAWAYS

The stigma, myths, and negative attitudes associated with breast cancer can make women afraid to admit they have cancer or even afraid to undergo routine screenings or ask their doctors about symptoms that are worrying them. Their silence, in turn, makes the stigma and myths even more potent, since there's little chance of the truth being revealed in time.

The best way to break free of the stigma, myths, and limiting beliefs and attitudes is to confront them and take needed action. Act by speaking up about breast cancer truths when you hear others believing or spreading misinformation and myths. Act by educating yourself, your family, and friends about the disease, which you are doing by reading this book. Act with courage by taking control of your own breasts and general health with routine screenings and preventative tools that can improve your well-being and give you peace of mind.

CHAPTER 8

BREAST CANCER RISK FACTORS AND PREVENTION

THE CAUSE OF BREAST CANCER is multifactorial, with multiple risk factors that combine to increase the likelihood of a woman being diagnosed with breast cancer during her lifetime. These causes can be divided into modifiable and non-modifiable risk factors.

The two biggest—and non-modifiable—risk factors for breast cancer are being of female gender and increasing age. Overall, the chances of developing cancer increase with age; this is why most breast cancer is diagnosed in the United States in women who are fifty years or older. However, in some developing countries like Nigeria, the data is pointing towards the development of breast cancer at an earlier age at diagnosis. This is yet to be established given the sparse data unavailable and limited cancer registries.

Over 70 percent of women who develop breast cancer have no risk factors aside from being of female gender and increasing age. Similarly, some women with multiple risk factors never develop breast cancer. This is why increased breast cancer awareness and screening is crucial—it's not possible to guess the odds, and the best way to be proactive is to arm yourself with knowledge and consult your healthcare provider frequently.

Let's take a deeper look into the modifiable and non-modifiable risk factors for breast cancer.

NON-MODIFIABLE RISK FACTORS
- Female gender
- Increasing age
- Genetic mutation: BRCA1, BRCA2, Li Fraumeni, Cowden syndrome. Genetic mutations like the BRCA genes make an individual at risk for breast and ovarian cancer.
- Family history
- Personal history
- High-risk breast lesions (atypical ductal hyperplasia, lobular hyperplasia)
- Breast density
- Radiation therapy at an early age (less than thirty years old)

Black women were included in the high-risk category group in the breast cancer screening guidelines issued in 2018 by the American College of Radiology (ACR) and Society for Breast Imaging (SBI) for the first time. This is due to the higher mortality rates from breast cancer in Black women (20 percent to 40 percent higher), despite similar occurrence rates of breast cancer among Black and white women. These differences can be attributed to tumor biology (Black women have a higher incidence of aggressive breast cancer subtypes), genetics, access to mammography, and differences in healthcare delivery patterns. They recommended:

> "All women, especially Black women and those of Ashkenazi Jewish descent, should be evaluated for breast cancer risk no later than age 30, so that those at higher risk can be identified and can benefit from supplemental screening."

MODIFIABLE RISK FACTORS
- Weight gain/obesity especially after menopause
- Sedentary lifestyle
- High fat and high carbohydrate diet

- Alcohol intake
- Smoking
- Combined hormonal replacement therapy (HRT): The use of hormonal therapy, especially after menopause, for more than five years increases your risk for breast cancer.

OBESITY AS A RISK FACTOR

Obesity is a chronic and complex medical condition associated with numerous health problems. It is a risk factor for metabolic syndrome, type 2 diabetes, and cardiovascular disease. It has a significant negative impact on morbidity and mortality outcomes. The estimated medical cost of obesity in the United States in 2019 was approximately $173 billion! Two out of three Americans (approximately 69 percent) are overweight or obese. Non-Hispanic Asian adults (17.4 percent) have the lowest rates compared to non-Hispanic Whites (42.2 percent). Non-Hispanic Blacks (49.6 percent) and Hispanic adults (44.8 percent) had higher rates, with non-Hispanic Black women having the highest rates of obesity overall at approximately 59 percent in the United States. Diet, physical activity, stress, genetics, and socioeconomic status contribute to the disparity of obesity in certain ethnic groups. Obesity is a definite twofer; it's linked to heart disease and breast cancer, the top two disease killers of women. We need to keep obesity in check, and here's why.

Obesity is an independent risk factor for breast cancer. It is the single most preventable risk factor for many diseases, including breast cancer. Studies have shown that body mass index (BMI) is an important predictor of cancer risk. According to the research done by GLOBOCAN International Agency for Research Cancer (IARC) in 2012, the percentage of breast cancer cases attributable to excess BMI in women worldwide was 33 percent. In April 2016, the IARC formed a working group to reassess the preventive effects of weight control on cancer risk. It concluded that the absence of excess body fat lowers the risk of most cancers.

The rapid rise of worldwide obesity has spurred an interest in understanding the links between obesity and diseases such as breast cancer, as well as in developing strategies to reduce the risk of breast cancer among people who are overweight or obese. Obesity is associated with an increased risk of estrogen receptor-positive postmenopausal breast cancer and worse cancer-related outcomes for all breast tumor subtypes. Obese breast cancer patients are also at increased risk for local recurrence. A review of scientific research showed a 35 percent to 40 percent increased risk of breast cancer recurrence and death independent of menopausal status. Compared to non-obese women with breast cancer, obese women are more likely to have surgical, chemotherapy, and radiation therapy complications. Abe et al. reported in the 1970s that obese breast cancer patients had larger infiltrative tumors at diagnosis, higher lymphatic and vascular invasion rates, and worse overall survival outcomes than their non-obese counterparts. Black breast cancer survivors are 70 percent more likely to be obese than white breast cancer survivors.

The complete biological mechanism of how obesity is linked to breast cancer is not fully known. However, biologically active adipose (fat) tissue is implicated. High levels of the aromatase enzyme in obese individuals cause an excess conversion of androgen to estrogen. Thus, there is an increase in estrogen receptor-positive breast cancer. Biological active fat tissue also produces proinflammatory mediators, contributing to triple-negative cancers, local and distant recurrence, and overall survival.

Obesity affects a woman's breast health trajectory from screening mammography habits to survival outcomes. For example, due to many factors such as access to care, health-seeking behaviors, socioeconomic status, and stigma related to obesity, obese women are less adherent to mammographic screening. Given the adverse effect of obesity on breast cancer development and outcomes, we need solutions on an individual and systemic level to treat obese patients with cancer. Conversations and interventions for preventing obesity from developing or progressing need to be front and center.

Research suggests that even small reductions in weight can have a significant impact on breast cancer risk. For example, a research study found that women who lost four to ten pounds had a 13 percent risk reduction in breast cancer than women with stable weight. This percentage rose to 16 percent in women who lost ten to twenty pounds, and to 25 percent in women who lost more than twenty pounds. The lead author of the study, Lauren Teras, PhD, noted that even a modest amount of sustained weight loss is associated with lower breast cancer risk for women over fifty. This is great news and a wonderful motivation to shed some unwanted excess weight.

I strongly encourage lifestyle changes with a healthy diet, increased physical activity, and mental health therapy as needed, such as cognitive behavioral therapy. However, depending on the situation, these may not be enough or yield consistent results for everyone. Speak to a doctor about medical and surgical options that help prevent obesity and alleviate associated diseases. It's a lifelong journey. You don't have to go it alone. Remember that even small steps pay dividends.

Definitions of Classes of Overweight and Obesity

Class	Body Mass Index (BMI) kg/m²
Overweight	**25.0–29.9**
Obesity	
Class 1	**30.0–34.9**
Class 2	**35.0–39.9**
Class 3	**>40.0**

BMI is a person's weight in kilograms (or pounds) divided by the square of height in meters (or feet).

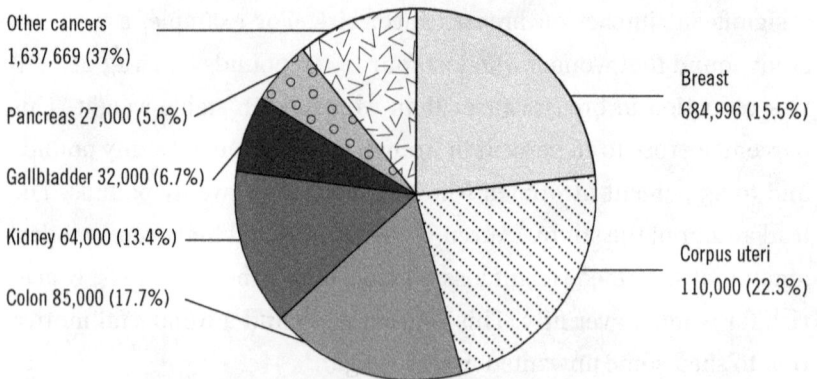
Cancer cases among both sexes attributable to excess BMI, worldwide in 2012

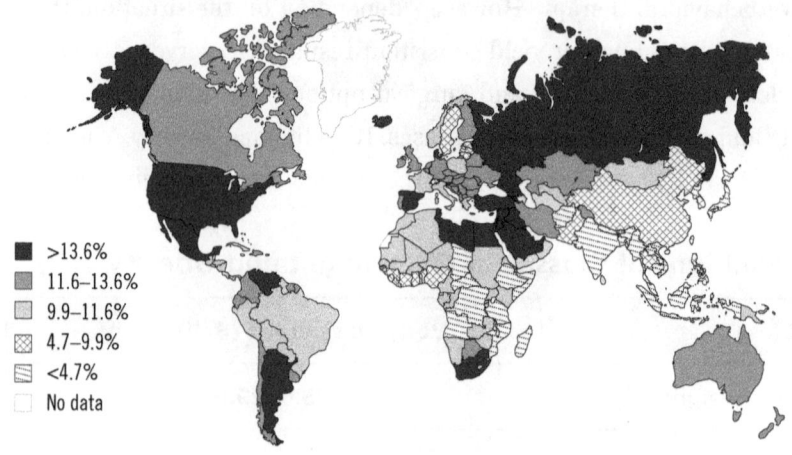
Fraction (%) of all postmenopausal breast cancer among females attributable to excess BMI, worldwide in 2012

MAIN TAKEAWAYS

Breast cancer risk encompasses both non-modifiable and modifiable risk factors. Increasing age and being female are the two highest risk factors for developing breast cancer and are non-modifiable. Other non-modifiable risk factors include genetics—personal or family history of breast cancer. However, modifiable risk factors such as smoking, alcohol consumption, physical activity levels, hormone replacement therapy, and reproductive history can also significantly influence risk. Lifestyle choices, which include regular screening, maintaining a healthy weight, limiting alcohol intake, and being mindful of hormonal influences, are key strategies to mitigating breast cancer risk. Understanding and addressing both non-modifiable and modifiable risk factors empowers you to take proactive steps in your breast health journey, facilitating early detection and improving overall outcomes.

CHAPTER 9
BREAST CANCER PREVENTION AND EARLY DETECTION

"BREAST HEALTH" CAN BE DEFINED as the correct functioning of the breasts and a lack of disease. Often the actions that help you to prevent breast cancer are also those that help you to detect it in the long term.

I, like most people, wish for a world in which cancer is nonexistent, and I pray for the day when cancer can be entirely prevented regardless of genetics.

Until that day, the first step in improving outcomes associated with breast cancer is to detect it in its earliest stages. Some studies have suggested that early detection can reduce breast cancer deaths by as much as 30 percent.

Here are some of the ways breast cancer can be detected early.

MONTHLY HABITS
Self-Exam
A breast self-exam is the simplest and cheapest method of finding lumps or other changes that may indicate the presence of cancer.

The best time to perform this exam is one to two weeks after your period if your periods are regular. If your periods are not regular, you can perform a self-exam the same date of every month.

BREAST SELF EXAMINATION

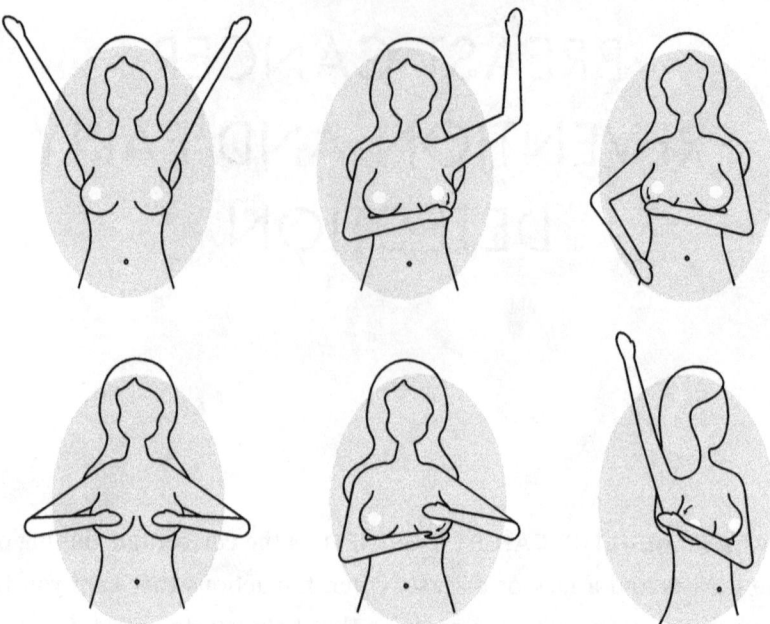

The exam should be performed once with your arm extended over your head and once with your arm hanging at your side. Working from the nipple out, gently feel your breast for any unusual bumps or lumps that could indicate a tumor.

Breast tissue is ordinarily lumpy, so doing a baseline exam immediately after a clinical exam by a doctor will help you learn what your breasts normally feel like when healthy.

Seek medical advice from your doctor if you notice any of these symptoms:

- Swelling, redness, or discoloration of your breast
- Itchy rash or soreness in the nipple area
- Puckering or dimpling of the skin or nipple
- Discharge from the nipple
- Persistent pain in one spot
- Changes in the shape or size of your breast
- Lump or "knot" in the breast or underarm area

SIGNS AND SYMPTOMS

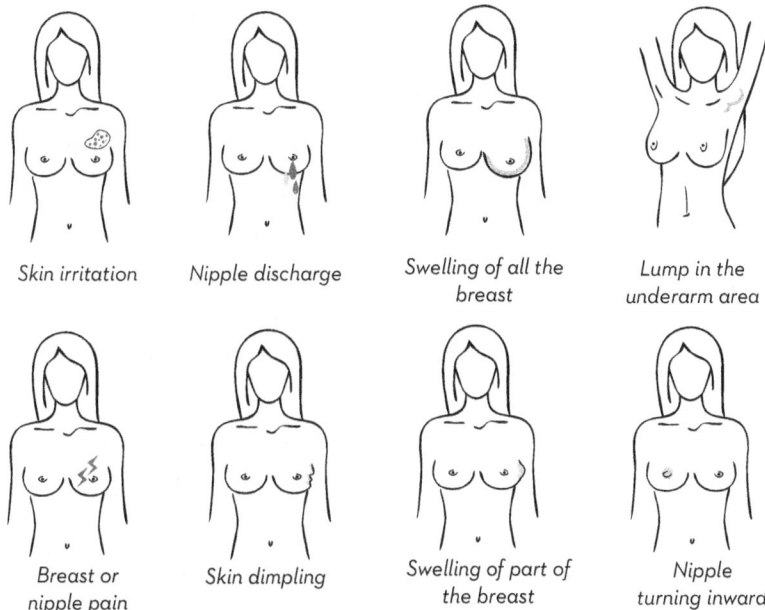

Skin irritation | Nipple discharge | Swelling of all the breast | Lump in the underarm area

Breast or nipple pain | Skin dimpling | Swelling of part of the breast | Nipple turning inward

Self-exams help you become more familiar with your breasts so you can feel changes more easily; however, they should not be used as a screening tool for breast cancer or as a substitute for regular screening exams, such as a mammography.

YEARLY HABITS

Clinical Exam

A clinical breast exam is performed by a doctor or other trained healthcare provider.

During the exam, your provider will feel your breasts and underarms to check for abnormalities while you're lying down and then perform a visual evaluation while you're sitting up.

A clinical breast exam is recommended for women over the age of twenty every three years, and annually for women over the age of forty. Typically for women over the age of forty, your doctor will often order a screening mammogram after the clinical exam.

Mammogram

A mammogram is a special X-ray used to generate a radiologic image of breast tissue.

As we described in previous chapters, during a mammogram, your breast is placed between the paddles of a mammogram unit, and light compression is used to keep the breast still and to generate a good-quality radiology image that can be used for the screening and diagnosis of breast diseases.

Mammography is currently the number-one imaging tool used for breast cancer detection in most patients. It can help find tumors that are too small to be felt by a patient or a doctor. Research studies have demonstrated a 30 percent decrease in mortality rates that can be attributed to early detection of breast cancer due to mammography.

In general, it is recommended that women over the age of forty have yearly mammograms. Women under the age of thirty usually are first evaluated with an ultrasound when they present with breast concerns. Mammograms are rarely performed on a woman under the age of twenty.

How to Prepare for a Mammogram

You may need a mammogram if you or your doctor have concerns or if you are getting a routine annual screening. On the day of your mammogram, a technologist who is specially trained in acquiring your images will ask questions about your personal and family history. You will be instructed to undress from the waist up, given a gown, and asked to wipe underneath your armpits. Deodorants and perfumes can cause artifacts on the mammogram that mimic cancer and can cause an unnecessary call back if present. A standard two images of each breast are acquired, with views from top to bottom and inner to outer for a typical screening mammogram. More images and views may be needed during a diagnostic mammogram evaluation. Your images will then be processed and sent to a radiologist (a doctor who specializes in interpreting medical images) for interpretation.

What Does My Mammogram Report Mean? BIRADS What?

Radiologists interpret mammograms using lexicon and guidelines from the Breast Imaging Reporting and Data System (BIRADS) atlas. The BIRADS atlas is a risk assessment and quality assurance tool developed by the American College of Radiology in 1992. It is now in its fifth edition released in December 2013. It is the standard used in breast imaging for terminology usage, report organization, and assessment structure. It provides a classification system for imaging modalities used in breast imaging—namely, mammography, ultrasound, MRI of the breast, and contrast enhanced mammography soon.

Birads Asssement/Recommendation

1: Negative for malignancy/Annual screening on schedule

2: Benign/Annual screening on schedule

3: Probably benign/Short-term follow-up (less than 2% chance of malignancy)

4: Suspicious malignancy/Biopsy recommended

5: Highly suspiciously malignancy/Biopsy recommended

6: Known biopsy proven malignancy/Follow-up as per oncology protocol

0: Additional imaging evaluation needed

The BIRADS assessment of your breast imaging report determines the next step of your management pathway. For example, BIRADS 1 and 2 indicate you can return to your annual breast screening schedule depending on your age and/or risk. BIRADS 3 indicates a probably benign finding that needs to be followed in one to six months depending on the findings and clinical symptoms. Typically, findings suspicious for an infection may require a short-term follow-up in four to six weeks after antibiotic therapy. A mass with benign characteristics such as fibroadenoma may be followed up every six months for a period of two years. If there are changes in symptoms or characteristics of the imaging findings that are suspicious, a biopsy will be performed. BIRADS 4 and 5 indicate suspicious to highly suspicious findings.

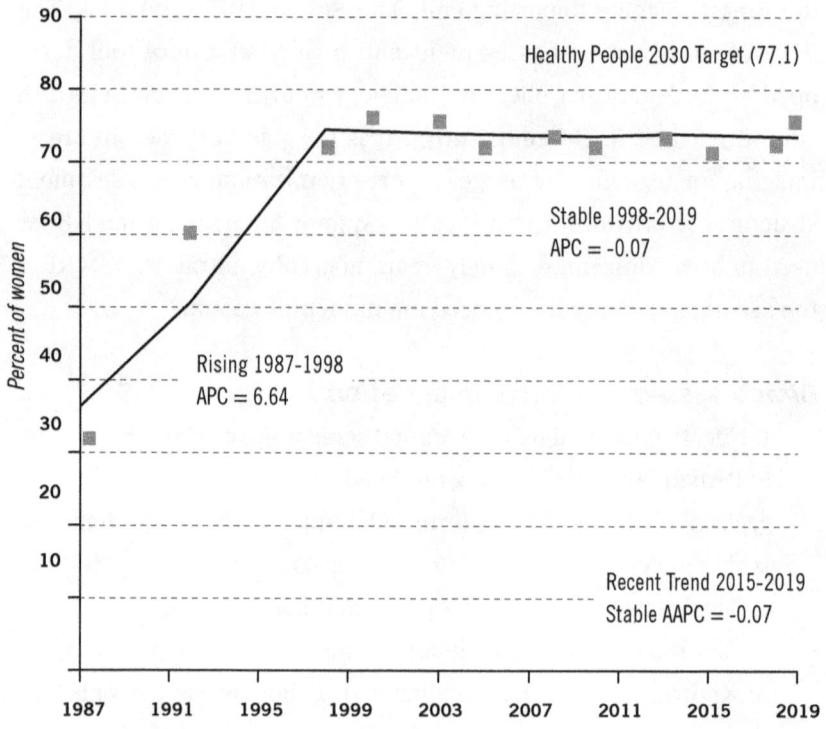

Source: Centers for Disease Control and Prevention, National Center for Health Statistics. Version 4.8 April 2020, National Cancer Institute. The AAPC is the Average Annual Percent Change and is based on the APCs calculated by Joinpoint. The Annual Percent Change (APC)/Average Annual Percent Change (AAPC) is statistically significant.

Debate about the Mammogram

Overdiagnosis and overtreatment are currently the main points of the controversy that surrounds screening mammography. Currently, our society places a higher value on early detection rather than late detection and thus potentially premature death. Hopefully, as medicine continues to advance, our detection tools will become more tailored and accurate. The one goal we can all agree on is the eradication of cancer in humanity once and for all. Until then, we use what is available to save lives to the best of our ability.

Compliance Rates for Mammography

According to the Centers for Disease Control (CDC), under the current guidelines, the compliance rate for mammography screening in 2019 for women ages fifty to seventy-four was 76.4 percent. There is concern that, if the guidelines are not clear or there is a large interval between screenings, compliance rates will decrease, with a resultant increase in mortality rates from breast cancer. This effect will be worse in women from lower-socioeconomic groups who have a lower compliance rate to begin with.

The downstream negative effects of the unprecedented COVID-19 pandemic on preventative health services such as screening mammograms also must be considered when regarding mortality and morbidity from delayed cancer diagnosis. In what has been described as one of the biggest disruptions to medical care in American history, screening and diagnostic mammograms came to an almost grinding halt for a significant portion of the first half of 2020, through the beginning and height of the pandemic. The severity of the consequences from the resultant delayed cancer diagnoses, the development/worsening of negative health-seeking behaviors, and the widening of previous health disparities is yet to be determined.

Thus, the importance of participating in a breast cancer screening mammogram at regular intervals cannot be overstated. It is highly recommended for women over the age of forty with average risk, and it is a must for women with high risk.

ULTRASOUND

"Ultrasound" is the name of the technology that uses sound waves to create images of breast tissue. It does not use radiation. It can be done in your doctor's office if they have the equipment, or at a hospital or a radiology center.

It is the second most common imaging tool used to image the breast. It is used to provide additional data following an abnormal mammogram.

It's especially useful for women with dense breast tissue, who can have lumps that a mammography may not detect. It is the first-line imaging tool in most practices for women under the age of thirty.

Diagnostic Ultrasound

A targeted or focused ultrasound is usually performed in the setting of a symptomatic patient who has an area of clinical concern and, most commonly, a lump. It may be performed in conjunction with a mammogram typically in patients over the age of thirty. Breast imaging evaluation of women under the age of thirty and pregnant women usually begins with a diagnostic ultrasound evaluation.

If a woman is called back from a screening mammogram due to a noncalcified finding such as a mass, architectural distortion, etc., she will also get a diagnostic ultrasound as part of her further evaluation.

Supplemental Whole-Breast Screening Ultrasound

Breast density is determined by several factors and can only be determined via mammography. Approximately 50 percent of women above the age of forty have dense breasts, and most women are unaware of the density of their breasts until they get a mammogram (which is usually at the beginning of their annual screenings, at the age of forty). Women with dense breasts have an increased risk of breast cancer. A limitation of mammography is the "masking effect" of cancer that can occur with dense breasts: dense breasts appear white on a mammogram, and so does cancer!

Quantitative volumetric breast density software can be used to assess the density of breast tissue on a mammogram. Radiologists can also use a subjective qualitative assessment to stratify breast density, which is currently the preferred method. It is based on the ratio of dense fibrous and glandular breast tissue relative to fatty tissue. Dense fibrous and glandular tissue is harder to evaluate on a mammogram. It is divided into four categories. A mammogram report may indicate a breast density statement:

A) The breast tissue is almost entirely fatty (0 to 25 percent dense tissue relative to fat).
B) Scattered fibro-glandular densities (25 to 50 percent).
C) Heterogeneous fibro-glandular density, which may obscure small masses (50 to 75 percent).
D) Extremely dense breast tissue, which limits the sensitivity of mammography (greater than 75 to 100 percent).

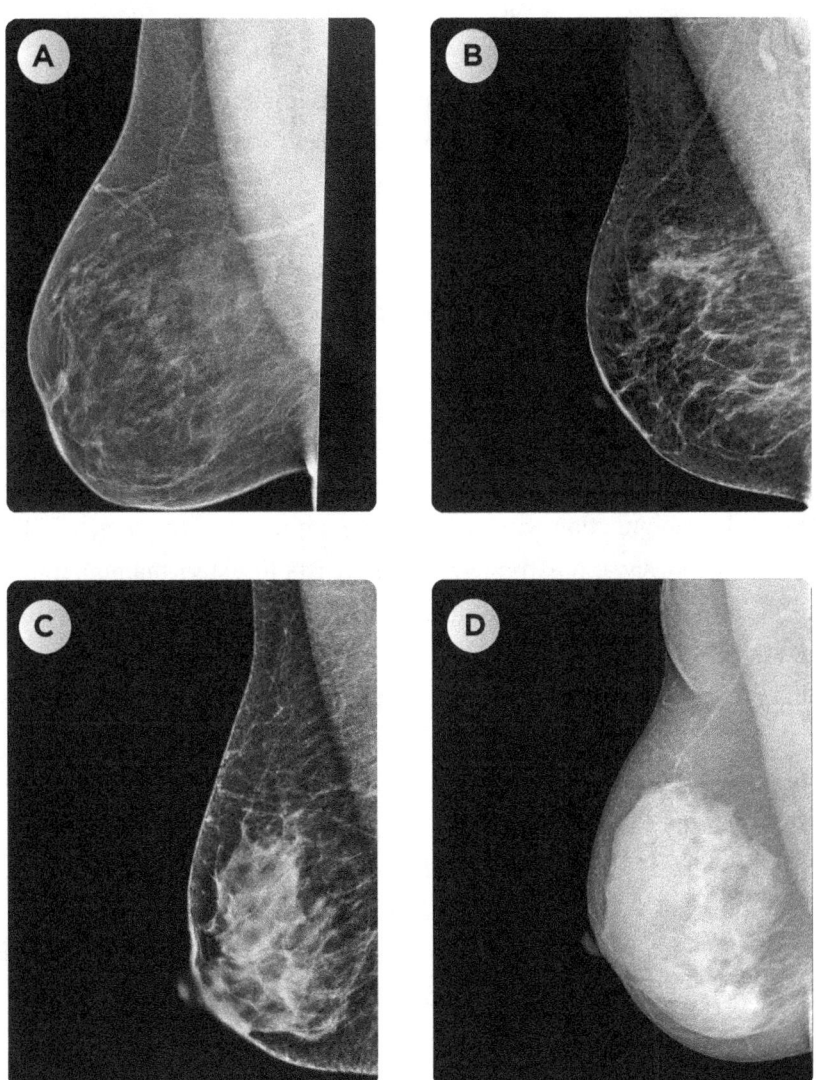

In the United States, all patients who get a mammogram must be notified of their breast density in a lay summary with language mandated by law. A mammogram report may have a statement like this example used by the American Cancer Society:

> *"Your mammogram shows that your breast tissue is dense. Dense breast tissue is common and is not abnormal. However, dense breast tissue can make it harder to evaluate the results of your mammogram and may also be associated with an increased risk of breast cancer. This information about the results of your mammogram is given to you so you will be informed when you talk with your doctor. Together, you can decide which screening options are right for you. A report of your results was sent to your primary physician."*
> *(American Cancer Society website)*

Due to breast density laws that require mammography reports to indicate the density of a woman's breasts, more women are becoming aware of their breast density. A supplemental ultrasound can be performed in conjunction with a screening mammogram for women with heterogeneously and extremely dense breasts to detect mammographically occult breast cancers. Currently, thirty-eight states in the United States now have some form of breast density notification laws, and some have expanded insurance coverage depending on the policy and plan.

There is some controversy as to whether all women with dense breasts—which is theoretically half of the screening population—should have knee-jerk whole breast screening ultrasounds, as there is an increased risk of *false positives* (i.e., findings that are detected, biopsied, and found not to be cancer). It depends on who you ask. A discussion with your doctor about the benefits and risks tailored to your personal history and risk factors will be helpful in making an informed decision.

MRI (Magnetic Resonance Imaging)

A breast MRI can be used to evaluate the extent of disease spread in women who have a new diagnosis of cancer, to assess treatment response, and to assist with surgical planning. It is also used as a screening examination for women who have a high risk of breast cancer. These are women who have greater than 20 percent lifetime risk of developing breast cancer.

For instance, women with first-degree relatives (mother, sister) with a premenopausal history of breast cancer or women known to have the breast cancer gene (BRCA1 or BRCA2) fall into this high-risk screening category.

Globally, not all women can afford or have access to a mammogram or ultrasound scan. This is where the practice of breast self-exams becomes important. This is often how breast cancer is detected by a woman, especially in a low-resource setting. Learn a breast self-exam technique that works for you, and commit yourself to carrying it out regularly. Don't stop there—spread the word, and empower other women around you also to become breast aware.

If you are at a high risk of developing breast cancer due to personal or family history or both, speak with your doctor about creating a customized breast cancer screening plan.

LONG-TERM CANCER PREVENTION
Lifestyle Modifications

One of the most common fears among women is breast cancer. It is important to understand that everything you eat, drink, and do daily may increase or decrease the risk of getting many cancers, including breast cancer. The risk of getting some cancers, breast cancer included, may be significantly reduced by merely living a healthier lifestyle. Eating a healthy diet, exercising regularly, and losing weight may help to reduce your chance of developing breast cancer. According to Johns Hopkins Medical Center, here are a few ways to practice breast cancer prevention:

- Stay within a healthy weight. The risk of breast cancer increases in women who are obese, especially after menopause.
- Eat healthy, which includes a diet high in fruit and vegetables, lean protein, and whole grains.
- Stay physically active with moderate exercise.
- Avoid or significantly limit the use of alcohol.
- Do not smoke.
- Breastfeed for as long as possible.
- Avoid using hormone replacement therapy following menopause.
- Get regular screenings for breast cancer.
- If you have a high risk of developing breast cancer, such as for genetic reasons, you should have extra screenings and talk with your doctor about estrogen-blocking drugs.

FOODS, NATURAL SUPPLEMENTS, AND BREAST CANCER
Foods

Research shows that our eating patterns have a significant influence on our overall health. A healthy diet also reduces our risk of developing different types of cancer, including breast cancer.

As mentioned above, following a diet that is rich in fruits, vegetables, and whole grains, and low in refined sugar, carbohydrates, and saturated fat, helps to reduce your risk of developing cancer.

There are no magical foods or teas that will remove your risk of breast cancer or other breast cancer issues—or cure breast cancer, for that matter. The key concept here is *eating patterns*, which is what you usually eat on a day-to-day basis. If you eat lots of spinach for dinner one day, you will boost your nutrient intake in the short term. Still, it will not reduce your risk of developing cancer unless you eat spinach, along with a variety of other fruits and vegetables, as part of your regular diet. The same goes for avoiding foods that may contribute to your health risk; if you eat a slice of cake once a month, it will generally not affect your health, but if you eat half a cake daily, it could affect your health status and your weight.

When grocery shopping, choose whole foods like fresh fruits and vegetables, whole grains, and lean proteins such as eggs, fish, beans, and chicken. Research has shown that women who have been diagnosed with early stage breast cancer may live longer when they eat a healthy diet that includes whole grains, healthy fats, lean protein, vegetables, and fruits. You can find a comprehensive list of foods you should aim to include in your diet regularly at Eat to Beat Cancer (eattobeat.org).

Natural Supplements

Although there are no magic bullets when it comes to natural supplements that could prevent breast cancer, there are several supplements that have natural cancer-fighting properties, which may be beneficial. These natural supplements include the following:

- **Flaxseeds**: Rich in omega-3 fats and rich in dietary fiber, flaxseeds may help to improve cholesterol levels. While you can take flaxseed oil as a supplement to benefit from the omega-3 fats, you can add whole or ground flaxseeds to smoothies and other foods to make the most of the protein and fiber contained in the husk.
- **Turmeric or curcuma**: This spice is best known for its powerful anti-inflammatory and antioxidant properties. Antioxidants help to scavenge free radicals that can damage cells and spur the development of cancer. If you don't want to take supplements, you can add turmeric to foods and drinks, or drink turmeric tea daily.
- **Bitter melon**: Also known as bitter gourd, bitter melon extract can help to reduce blood sugar, and it may decrease cholesterol levels. It also contains chemicals that initial studies have shown have the potential to kill cancer cells. If you can buy the whole fruit, you'll find it is delicious and versatile.
- **Fish oil**: Fish oil is high in unsaturated fats, which is a good choice for a healthy diet. If you are looking to supplement with fish oil, find a brand that is high in omega-3 fatty acids, rather than omega-6 fatty acids.

- **Saw palmetto extract**: Some initial studies show that saw palmetto may help to inhibit the proliferation of breast cancer cells.
- **Vitamin D**: Research suggests that women who have low levels of vitamin D are at higher risk of developing breast cancer. Since Black women have more melanin in their skin, they tend to be more at risk of being deficient in vitamin D.
- **CoQ10**: Several studies have shown that CoQ10 supplementation's antioxidant power has the potential to increase the immune system response to breast cancer.

One of the most beneficial supplements that may aid in helping to prevent breast cancer is omega-3 acids, which are essential for blocking inflammation and encouraging cell growth. Salmon and sardines typically contain high levels of omega-3 fatty acids.

Regardless of the health benefits of supplements you read about, it is important that you **talk about supplementation with your healthcare provider before starting a supplement regimen.** This is especially true if you are pregnant, planning on becoming pregnant, breastfeeding, or if you have a history of breast cancer or other forms of cancer. Supplements interact with everyone differently, so medical advice is important.

Also remember that diet is just one piece of the puzzle when it comes to breast cancer risk. There are factors involved in the risk of developing breast cancer that cannot be controlled, such as family history, being of the female gender, and increasing age. The most important aspect of prevention is to be thoroughly diligent in taking all precautions possible. If you are overweight, talk with your doctor about a recommended weight-loss regimen.

CHEMOPREVENTION

Chemoprevention is the use of drugs to reduce the risk of cancer.

The drugs tamoxifen and raloxifene can be used to help lower breast cancer risk in certain women. These drugs block the action of estrogen in breast tissue. Raloxifene is only used in women who have gone through menopause, while tamoxifen can be used in women even if they haven't gone through menopause.

Experts recommend that these drugs only be used to lower breast cancer risk in women who are *known* to be at increased risk of the disease. These drugs can also have some side effects, so it's important to understand the possible benefits and risks of taking one of the drugs.

Other drugs are being studied to see if they can lower the risk of breast cancer.

The American Cancer Society website has more information on the possible benefits and risks of chemopreventive drugs.

PROPHYLACTIC MASTECTOMY

A prophylactic mastectomy is a surgery where breast tissue is removed completely before cancerous tissue is detected. It is an elective surgery for women who have a very high risk of developing breast cancer.

The word *prophylactic* means that it is a preventative surgery, and it can reduce the risk of developing breast cancer by up to 97 percent. It doesn't eliminate the risk entirely, because some breast tissue is left behind with a minimal but residual risk of developing into cancer.

Prophylactic mastectomies are also an option for women who have or have had cancer in one breast and choose to have the other breast removed to reduce the risk of a second breast cancer diagnosis. A prophylactic mastectomy may be recommended with the following scenarios:

- Genetic mutations such as BRCA1, BRCA2, etc. Over seventy new genetic mutations have been linked to cancer (CHEK2, PTEN, ATM, PALB2, TP53 etc.).
- A strong family history of breast cancer.
- Personal history of breast cancer.

MAIN TAKEAWAYS

A mainstay of risk reduction for any disease, including cancer, is engagement in positive lifestyle changes, which includes a proper nutritional diet and regular exercise. Avoiding tobacco products and limiting alcohol intake are also essential lifestyle modifications. Most importantly, see your healthcare provider regularly for routine physical exams, and develop a customized cancer screening plan based on your age and risk factors.

CHAPTER 10

BREAST CANCER DIAGNOSIS AND TREATMENT JOURNEY

IF A CLINICAL BREAST EXAM, mammography, or other imaging study reveals an unusual mass inside your breast that your healthcare provider feels may be cancer, the next step usually involves taking a small sample (biopsy) of the tissue comprising the lump and studying it under a microscope.

A biopsy is considered the "gold standard" when it comes to cancer diagnosis. It involves the removal of tissue from the body for examination to detect the presence or absence of disease. It is usually performed in one of two ways: surgically or with a needle.

SURGICAL BIOPSY

For this approach, your doctor or healthcare provider will make a small incision in your breast to remove the suspected tumor so that it may be studied. Although it's the most accurate form of breast cancer diagnosis, it's also the most invasive because it involves making a larger incision that may leave a scar. It usually also requires sedation or general anesthesia. Surgical excisional biopsies allow for examination of the entire mass as well as surrounding tissue to assess the extent of disease.

NEEDLE BIOPSY

Needle biopsies are far less invasive than surgical biopsies and tend to be the preferred method for initial diagnosis in most cases. A hollow

9-gauge to 25-gauge needle is used for tissue sampling. There are two ways to perform needle biopsies: core needle and fine needle.

PERCUTANEOUS CORE NEEDLE BIOPSY

Core needle biopsies can be performed for palpable and non-palpable masses. Most palpable masses can be biopsied in your doctor's office using a small amount of local anesthetic to numb the area. For non-palpable masses, the procedure is a little more involved and will probably need to be done in a medical center, hospital, or clinic, where image guidance such as an ultrasound or mammography can be used to guide the placement of the needle.

FINE NEEDLE ASPIRATION

A fine needle biopsy uses a thinner needle than core needle biopsy, and it is only used when a mass is palpable. It is often used as a quick method of sampling breast tissue after a clinical exam reveals a suspicious area. A fine needle biopsy is less uncomfortable than a core needle biopsy; however, because it is so delicate and thin, there is a risk the needle will miss the finding and collect healthy tissue, resulting in a false negative and a delay in treatment. It also requires the expedient presence of a cytopathologist (a doctor trained in the diagnosis of human diseases by the study of cells), which is not always readily available at most health centers.

The type of biopsy performed is typically based on your clinical profile, as well as the results of your clinical breast exam and the imaging findings on your mammography, ultrasound, and/or MRI. Most commonly, needle biopsies are performed first, followed by a surgical removal based on the results. A needle biopsy prior to surgical removal allows for an algorithmically evidence-based approach to diagnosis, especially if the results yield a malignancy. Immunohistochemistry can be obtained on the sample to find out the receptors of the tumor, which will help to better tailor treatment. Tumor receptors are proteins found on the surface of cancer cells or within the cells. They play a crucial role in how cancer cells grow and spread. In breast cancer, the most common receptors tested for are estrogen receptors (ER), progesterone receptors (PR), and human epidermal growth factor receptor 2 (HER2). Testing for these receptors helps determine the type of breast cancer and guides treatment decisions, as different receptors respond to different therapies.

Finally, it's important to understand that a biopsy will not cause your cancer to spread. In fact, a biopsy is the best way to make sure that a lump that turns out to be cancer is appropriately diagnosed and treated. It provides essential information about the type of cancer so your oncology team can determine the best course of treatment for you.

I'VE HAD MY BIOPSY—WHAT'S NEXT? THE MANAGEMENT PATHWAY

After a breast biopsy has been performed, it is important that a radiologic and pathology (rad path) correlation be performed by the radiology department to help direct further management.

Benign: No malignancy or atypical findings. Depending on the patient's age, symptoms, and history, a patient will return for annual screening on schedule, or for a short-term follow-up to ensure stability. There are some benign lesions, such as cellular fibroepithelial lesions and phyllodes, that are recommended for surgical excision due to their propensity for rapid growth.

High-risk: There are certain lesions that are noncancerous but considered high risk, meaning that their presence increases the risk for breast malignancy not necessarily in that lesion but in that patient. Depending on the institutions and their protocol, a surgical excision or close follow-up imaging surveillance is performed. In some cases, the patient is recommended to have additional screening with breast magnetic resonance imaging (MRI).

Atypical: Atypical cells in a biopsy specimen indicate that a suspicious change is happening. Biopsy results with atypia are watched closely or sent for surgical excision. In the case of atypical ductal hyperplasia (overgrowth of cells lining the milk ducts), for instance, the upstage to ductal carcinoma in situ (abnormal cells lining a milk duct but that haven't spread beyond it into the surrounding breast tissue) can be as high as 30 percent or more.

Discordant: The pathology results may not correlate with the image findings. This happens rarely, but is the reason why a radiology-pathology correlation is important—in the rare event of a false-negative result. For example, a spiculated mass on mammogram and ultrasound comes back as fibrocystic changes or a fibroadenoma. In this case, the pathology results will be deemed discordant from the radiologic image findings. A re-biopsy can be performed, or the patient is sent for surgical excision.

Malignant: The pathology results identified invasive cancer cells. The grade of malignancy, Grades 1 to 3, is often included in the pathology report. Immunochemistry (IHC) is also performed to identify the molecular subtype of the cancer based on the receptors being expressed (if any) by the tumor—that is, estrogen, progesterone, or human epidermal receptor growth factor (HER-2). There are five molecular subtypes of breast cancer based on the combination of genes being expressed. The combination of receptor expression determines the behavior of the cancer. An ER+/PR+ is considered very treatable and less aggressive than triple negative cancer (ER-/PR-/HER2).

1. Luminal A: (ER+/PR+/HER2-)
2. Luminal B: (ER+/PR-/HER2-)
3. Luminal B-like: (ER+/PR-/HER2+)
4. HER-2 enriched: (ER-/PR-/HER2+)
5. Triple negative or basal cell: (ER-/PR-/HER-2). This is seen in Black women, women with BRCA1 mutation, and young women.

BREAST CANCER TREATMENT OPTIONS

Breast cancer is treated in a multidisciplinary manner with several treatment options based on the patient's health, age, type, and extent of disease. Types of breast cancer treatment include the following.

Breast Surgery

This involves removal of the tumor and checking of the sentinel lymph nodes under the arm to assess for metastasis.

Breast Conservation Surgery

This approach removes the tumor, ensuring the margins of the resected tissue have no tumor. A significant amount of unaffected breast tissue remains.

A lumpectomy or partial mastectomy removes the tumor along with a small amount of surrounding tissue to ensure negative margins. In some cases, patients undergo neoadjuvant chemotherapy to reduce the size of a large tumor to see if breast conservation is feasible.

Mastectomy

A simple mastectomy removes the entire breast. A modified radical mastectomy removes the breast, the lymph nodes under the arm, and the tissue that separates the breast from the chest muscles. In some cases, part of the muscle may be removed. A mastectomy may be followed by reconstruction surgery using implants. Implants may be with silicone or flap (fat transfer from elsewhere in the body) reconstruction.

Sentinel Lymph Node Biopsy Followed by Surgery

A sentinel node is the first lymph node to receive drainage from a tumor, which makes it the most likely place for cancer to spread. During a sentinel node biopsy, a dye is used to track drainage from the tumor, and the first node to receive the dye is removed. The node tissue is examined under a microscope to determine whether more lymph nodes need to be removed. Following the biopsy, the tumor is surgically removed.

Radiation Therapy
Radiation therapy uses high-intensity X-rays or other types of radiation to kill cancer cells and prevent them from spreading. External radiation uses radiation from a machine directed at the tumor; internal radiation uses radioactive substances sealed in small devices that are implanted near the tumor. These devices release radiation over time directly to the tumor.

Chemotherapy
Chemotherapy uses drugs to kill cancer cells or stop their growth and development. Chemotherapy drugs may be taken by mouth or injected directly into the bloodstream to enable them to reach cancer cells anywhere in the body. Drugs may also be injected directly into the cancerous area. Chemotherapy may be given prior to surgery and radiation as neoadjuvant therapy, or after surgery and radiation to kill any residual cancer cells as adjuvant therapy.

Hormonal Therapy
About two-thirds of breast cancer have hormone receptors of estrogen and progesterone. Hormonal therapy or endocrine therapy targets these receptors, which inhibit or slow down the growth of the tumor. They are anti-estrogen and stop estrogen production by your body. Hormonal therapy can also be used as chemoprevention to lower risk. Aromatase inhibitors (i.e., anastrozole) or selective estrogen receptor modulators (SERMs, i.e., tamoxifen) are typically used. Usually, a patient is on hormonal therapy for at least five years.

Targeted and Immune Therapy
Targeted therapy are drugs used to target specific parts of tumor cells, such as proteins and receptors. They usually have less effect on non-cancerous cells. A common targeted therapy in breast cancer treatment is with the drug trastuzumab (Herceptin). It targets the HER-2 receptor, which signals tumor cells to grow and divide. Targeted therapies

are relatively new and cannot be used for all types of cancers. Immune therapy uses your immune system to fight breast cancer cells directly, indirectly by boosting your immune system, or by tagging the cancer cells for better identification by other drugs.

MAIN TAKEAWAYS

It is important to remember that with breast cancer diagnosis and treatment, early detection saves lives, and a comprehensive approach tailored to each individual is essential. From initial screening to diagnosis and treatment, it is crucial to prioritize both medical expertise and emotional support. While receiving a breast cancer diagnosis can be overwhelming, it is important to remember that you are not alone. Numerous treatment options are available, including surgery, chemotherapy, radiation therapy, and targeted therapies tailored to each situation. Throughout the journey, maintaining open communication with your healthcare team, seeking support from loved ones, and accessing resources such as support groups can provide comfort and strength. With proper support and treatment, there is hope for a brighter future beyond breast cancer.

CHAPTER 11
SURVIVORSHIP: BEYOND THE DIAGNOSIS

When we are no longer able to change a situation—
we are challenged to change ourselves.
—Viktor E. Frankl

THE ONLY CONSTANT IS CHANGE, and a moment that changes a life forever is a cancer diagnosis. I have witnessed this imminent change as it approached the lives of women in my clinical practice. I have seen the tension, uncertainty, and fear on my patients' faces when I have informed them they need a biopsy for a finding. Even as I tell them this, I know the results will be cancer and it will become the harbinger of the looming life change ahead. My patients can often sense this knowledge, but they remain hopeful for the results. Sadly, nothing can prepare anyone for the tsunami of change brought by the words, "I'm so sorry, but unfortunately, your biopsy results came back as cancer."

For some, it is their worst fears realized and a wake-up call that inspires positive life change. For others, the diagnosis overpowers them so negatively that, even in remission, they never truly recover from the emotional and physical blow. A close call where a biopsy turned out benign, or a breast cancer diagnosis of a close friend or family member, can also be a trigger for positive change. No matter what the catalyst is, change is hard! It comprises a mindset shift and a physical, mental, emotional, and spiritual reset.

Each woman's treatment experience is unique, and what is considered "normal" is different for everyone. There is no one-size solution for the next phase after treatment—"the rest of your life." Breast cancer survivors, their loved ones, and caregivers must always consider this. The perspective of each breast cancer survivor is unique. Survivorship for some begins when treatment for the current breast cancer diagnosis—that is, surgery, chemoradiation therapy, etc.—is complete. For others, it starts from the moment of diagnosis, which is also what the National Cancer Institute notes. Regardless of one's definition of when survivorship begins, the journey to start living an integrated and healthy lifestyle that promotes wholeness becomes a priority. Once treatment is complete, life is never the same again. After seemingly endless medical appointments, a rollercoaster of emotions, a side-effect-ridden body, and an out-of-whack sense of self, identity, and belonging, it is time for the "rest of my life" phase. Questions and fears arise: about the risk of cancer coming back, a new cancer developing elsewhere in the body, how their medication interacts with other chronic medications, the short- and long-term side effects, navigating medical follow-ups, and the new limitations and restrictions on their life.

How does one lead the rest of their new life? Transitioning from a cancer diagnosis and cancer treatment to a return to "normal" living can feel like an emergence from a bottomless dark pit. How exactly does one go back to living a "normal" life after the grueling diagnosis and treatment journey of breast cancer? This chapter addresses the transition from life before cancer to life after cancer.

POST-TREATMENT SURVEILLANCE

As breast cancer is a common female malignancy and has a good prognosis when detected early, it is natural that there will be millions of breast cancer survivors. In the United States alone, there are more than four million breast cancer survivors. The health, well-being, and quality of life concerns after the initial treatment of breast cancer are important issues that must be addressed. The treatment journey for some breast cancer patients on hormonal therapy, for instance, can last up to ten years. Medical surveillance, short- and long-term side-effect management, and psychosocial and spiritual support are therefore important for the wellness of breast cancer survivors and should be approached holistically.

The National Comprehensive Cancer Network (NCCN) and American Cancer Society/American Society of Clinical Oncology (ACS/ASCO) breast cancer survivorship guides are good resources for evidence-based research and recommendations related to a person's breast cancer post-treatment journey.

BREAST CANCER-RELATED LYMPHEDEMA (BCRL)

The accumulation of lymphatic fluid in the soft tissues of the upper extremity is a commonly feared complication of breast cancer treatment. It affects approximately one in five women treated for breast cancer, and symptoms usually present within the first two years of treatment. Extensive interventions, such as a radical mastectomy, axillary dissection, and axillary radiation therapy, increase the risk of lymphedema. (At the time of surgery to remove breast cancer, the lymphatic drainage is evaluated to check for local metastasis through a procedure called a sentinel lymph node injection. See chapter 10. At times, a complete axillary dissection is performed, and the lymph nodes are removed. In addition, radiation therapy could also be performed in the axillary region. All these procedures have the potential for causing a problem with lymphatic drainage, which can lead to lymphedema.) A high body mass index (BMI) over 30kg/m2 is also a risk factor for developing BCRL.

Symptoms of lymphedema can vary from pain, numbness, and tingling to a swollen and heavy arm, which can decrease mobility and severely decrease daily function. Awareness, prevention, and early treatment of lymphedema is crucial. Pre-treatment education, skin care, exercises, compression garments, lymphatic drainage massages, and complete decongestion therapy are some of the ways to help prevent and manage lymphedema.

The approach for intervention has moved from an impairment-based model of reported and clinically evident limb swelling to one of a preventative protective screening approach. Patient self-reporting, limb-size measurements, perometry, and bioimpedance spectroscopy (BIS) are ways to measure and assess BCRL. For example, the L-Dex device is a tool that can be used during follow-up medical visits to screen for lymphedema by detecting an early buildup of fluid. This allows for early detection of lymphedema and opportunity for prompt intervention that hopefully will curb its progression.

BREAST, ARMPIT, CHEST, AND SHOULDER PAIN

Scars and keloids that develop after surgery can be treated with silicone creams and patches, cryotherapy, laser, and direct steroid injections. Numbness, tingling, and swelling are common after most surgeries, including lumpectomies and mastectomies. I have had patients come to me to evaluate the lumpectomy or mastectomy site for pain, puffiness, swelling, lumps, tenderness, pressure, twitching, pulling, etc. These symptoms are usually due to expected evolving changes after surgery due to the regeneration of nerves, absorption of fluid, and the body working on healing itself. Sometimes lumps occur from a postsurgical fluid collection (i.e., seroma) or fat necrosis. The workup for lumps after surgery is typically benign, but each lump still needs to be evaluated to rule out residual or recurrent cancer.

Depending on the type of axillary surgery and how extensive it was, a patient may develop axillary web syndrome (AWS) a few weeks or even years after surgery. AWS is common and reported to occur in a significant number of patients who have an axillary dissection. In AWS, single or multiple tight cords develop in the soft tissue of the operated armpit. The cords extend down the inner part of the upper arm, toward the elbow or the outer parts of the chest. These cords can be painful and limit the outward lifting of the upper arm. Progressive arm exercises, myofascial release massage techniques, manual lymphatic drainage, acupuncture, and other rehabilitative tools can help to alleviate pain and improve mobility after axillary surgery.

HAIR, SKIN, AND NAILS

The integumentary system—which comprises the skin (epidermis, dermis, hypodermis), sebaceous glands, hair, and nails—can be hit hard during cancer treatment. The skin is the largest body organ and plays a vital role in functioning as a barrier from harmful external elements. It is also crucial for heat and temperature regulation and vitamin D synthesis. Hair loss, changes in skin pigmentation, redness, swelling, dryness/flakiness, peeling, and increased sun sensitivity are some of the side effects that can occur with breast cancer treatment. Nails may become dry, brittle, and even fall off during therapy. Hydrating is essential, and so is the use of sunscreen and moisturizers; gentle products are encouraged. Hair loss is another side effect of treatment, which can be harsh on women who identify with their hair. Wigs, hats, and new haircuts could help weather the storm during treatment and when hair starts to grow back. Regrowth can take six months to one year. Some women report a difference in texture, color, and volume. Scalp hypothermia (cooling) can prevent or limit chemotherapy-induced alopecia (hair loss) due to breast cancer treatment. The scalp can be cooled with a cap or a scalp cooling system before, during, and after treatment. The cold temperature constricts the scalp's blood vessels and reduces the effects of chemotherapy on the scalp. The DigniCap, Paxman, and Amma systems are Federal Drug Agency (FDA) approved cooling systems in the United States.

OSTEOPOROSIS

Osteoporosis is a medical condition where the bones become more susceptible to fractures due to a weakened structure from decreased bone density. It's a concern for many people, including those undergoing breast cancer treatment.

Several factors can increase a person's risk of developing osteoporosis. These include age, gender (women are more likely to develop osteoporosis than men), family history, low calcium, poor vitamin D intake, smoking, excessive alcohol consumption, and certain medical conditions. Treatment for breast cancer can also increase a person's risk of developing osteoporosis. Certain chemotherapy drugs and hormone therapies, such as aromatase inhibitors, can decrease bone density and increase the risk of fractures.

It's essential for people who have been diagnosed with breast cancer to talk to their healthcare provider about their risk of developing osteoporosis and to take steps to protect their bone health. This includes making lifestyle changes such as regularly exercising, quitting smoking, reducing alcohol consumption, and consuming a balanced diet rich in calcium and vitamin D. People with breast cancer may need to take calcium and vitamin D supplements to help maintain their bone health. Weight-bearing exercises, walking, running, and weightlifting can also help build and maintain strong bones.

In addition to lifestyle changes, medication and other treatments may be recommended to manage osteoporosis. Bisphosphonates and denosumab (a human monoclonal antibody) are two medications commonly used to prevent and treat osteoporosis. These medications work by slowing the breakdown of bone tissue, and they can help to improve bone density and reduce the risk of fractures.

Women undergoing breast cancer treatment may be referred for a dual X-ray absorptiometry (DEXA) scan to monitor their bone health. With proper care and support, many people can maintain strong and healthy bones, even in the face of challenges related to breast cancer and its treatment.

BONE PAIN

Bone pain is a common symptom experienced by breast cancer patients, particularly those undergoing chemotherapy, radiation therapy, and hormone therapy. It can occur when cancer spreads to the bones. Bone pain can also develop or be the effect of various diseases and activities. Therefore, working with your healthcare provider is crucial for proper and effective management.

Managing bone pain can be challenging, but several treatment options are available. Pain relief medications, such as nonsteroidal anti-inflammatory drugs (NSAIDs), opioids, and medications that increase bone density like bisphosphonates, can help alleviate pain and reduce the risk of bone fractures.

Gentle exercises, such as walking or yoga, can help improve bone strength and reduce pain. Heat therapy, such as warm baths or heating pads, can also help relieve pain and stiffness.

CARDIAC TOXICITY

Breast cancer treatment with chemotherapy, radiation therapy, and other therapies can sometimes cause damage to the heart, leading to cardiac toxicity. Cardiac toxicity can range from mild, asymptomatic changes in heart function to severe, life-threatening conditions.

Chemotherapy drugs, such as anthracyclines and HER2-targeted agents, are among the most common culprits of cardiac toxicity. Anthracyclines, including doxorubicin and epirubicin, are effective drugs for treating breast cancer. Still, they can also cause damage to the heart muscle. HER2-targeted agents, such as trastuzumab and pertuzumab, can also lead to cardiac toxicity by interfering with the function of the heart muscle.

Radiation therapy, mainly when it involves the left breast, can also cause damage to the heart. This can lead to conditions such as cardiomyopathy, a heart muscle disease that can cause heart failure.

The risk of cardiac toxicity depends on several factors, including the type and dose of treatment, the patient's age, pre-existing heart conditions, and other medical factors. Older patients and those with pre-existing heart conditions are at higher risk of developing cardiac toxicity.

Symptoms of cardiac toxicity can include shortness of breath, fatigue, chest pain, palpitations, and swelling in the feet and ankles.

Diagnostic tests such as an echocardiography or a cardiac MRI assess heart function if cardiac toxicity is suspected.

Preventing cardiac toxicity when designing breast cancer treatment plans is essential. Strategies for reducing the risk of cardiac toxicity may include:

- Using lower doses of chemotherapy or radiation therapy.
- Using fewer toxic drugs to the heart.
- Carefully monitoring heart function throughout treatment.

Patients with cardiac toxicity related to treatment are monitored for long-term effects on heart function. This may involve regular echocardiography or other diagnostic tests to assess heart function and detect changes early. By carefully monitoring heart function and reducing the risk of cardiac toxicity, healthcare providers can ensure that patients receive the best care for their breast cancer.

SEXUAL INTIMACY

Long-term sexual dysfunction is common in women who have undergone breast cancer treatment, with some studies indicating as high as 80 percent of women who have been treated for breast cancer reporting sexual dysfunction.

During treatment, a woman is literally busy trying to survive; sexual intimacy naturally takes a back seat. Unfortunately, sexual activity doesn't go back to business as usual even after the acute phase of treatment. Side effects of therapy, decreased self-confidence due to new body image, weight fluctuations, menopausal symptoms (vaginal dryness, painful sexual intercourse), fatigue, stress, depression, anxiety, and a slew of other factors related to treatment may result in a low libido, desire, and sex drive.

How treatment will affect sexual health should be part of the breast cancer care plan. A lot of therapies used in the treatment of breast cancer can hinder sexual function one way or another. For example, a mastectomy causes a loss of sensation on the skin and nipples. This side effect should be discussed, in addition to cosmetic outcomes. Chemotherapy and hormonal therapy can cause vaginal dryness and a low sex drive. Primary-care physicians and oncologists may not broach the topic of sexual side effects or may not go into much detail. Experts such a sex therapist, pelvic floor therapists, and sexologists can be consulted sooner in the treatment process for proactivity and better management of side effects related to sexual health. Sex after breast cancer is possible!

BODY IMAGE

A woman's breast is not necessarily her identity, but it is a noticeable part of her, like her face. A female's breast goes through many stages, at puberty, during menstruation, pregnancy, lactation, and so on, so much so that we have different bras to help handle each stage. As expected, surgery and radiation therapy will create scars and post-treatment changes despite best efforts to achieve good cosmesis. The remnant of these procedures, most notably scars, thickening, asymmetry, and hyperpigmentation, can make a woman feel disfigured and feel unlike herself.

Breast cancer treatment can be perceived to strip away parts of the body that make a woman feel feminine. For instance, some women may undergo the entire gamut of therapy of bilateral mastectomy, bilateral oophorectomy (removal of ovaries), hair loss, and skin changes from chemo and radiation, to the extent that they may no longer recognize themselves on the other side of treatment.

MENOPAUSAL SYMPTOMS

Vaginal dryness and atrophy are common symptoms from breast cancer treatment, especially when hormonal therapy in the form of anti-estrogen medications (i.e., aromatase) is used. Vaginal lubricators, dilators, or laser therapy can help with these symptoms.

FERTILITY AND PREGNANCY

Leuorlide (Lupron) shuts down ovaries and can protect your eggs during treatment (as chemotherapy can be harmful for them). Pregnancy after breast cancer does not increase your risk of recurrence. It is safe to get pregnant and breastfeed your child when that moment comes.

WEIGHT FLUCTUATIONS

Breast cancer treatment, including chemotherapy, hormonal therapy, and radiation therapy, can result in weight changes for survivors. Chronic pain, fatigue, and mental health issues may also contribute to weight issues. Fluctuations in weight—usually flip-flopping from weight gain to weight loss—are common frustrating side effects of treatment.

Survivors who experience weight gain may be concerned about their self-esteem, appearance, and the impact on their overall health. Weight loss can be just as concerning, especially if it is significant, sudden, and unintended.

In some cases, weight changes may be related to the side effects of medication, which can cause disturbances and changes in metabolism. A healthy integrated lifestyle, which includes proper nutrition, regular exercise, and stress management, can help manage weight changes. Survivors can work with nutritionists, dietitians, fitness experts, and other specialists to develop a cancer rehabilitation plan. In addition, counseling or therapy can address emotional concerns related to weight changes.

It is important to remember that weight changes are a common breast cancer treatment side effect and can be managed with proper support and care. Discussing weight changes with healthcare providers is essential, so timely interventions can be initiated. With time and patience, survivors can work with their healthcare providers to find the right approach customized to their needs and goals.

MENTAL HEALTH

In addition to physical side effects of being a breast cancer survivor, there are also psychological burdens to consider. These may extend even beyond the active treatment or exacerbate known emotional and mental disorders.

Anxiety

Anxiety after a breast cancer diagnosis and during treatment is common; it occurs frequently and understandably. Feelings of worry, nervousness, and unease about the diagnosis and treatment journey are usually due to uncertainty, the fear of outcomes, and potential for recurrence. Anxiety may also manifest with physical symptoms, such as chest pain, shortness of breath, and gastrointestinal distress. Breast cancer patients may experience anxiety throughout their diagnosis, treatment, and recovery.

Several intervention strategies exist to help manage anxiety in breast cancer patients. These may include talk therapy and relaxation techniques, such as meditation or deep breathing exercises. Cognitive-behavioral therapy (CBT), a form of talk therapy, can be effective in helping patients change negative thought patterns that may be triggering and causing anxiety. Complementary therapies, such as acupuncture and massage therapy, may also help. These therapies have been shown to have a calming effect and can help promote relaxation. In some cases, medications such as benzodiazepines and antidepressants may also be prescribed to help manage anxiety symptoms.

Depression

Depression is a common and severe mood disorder that can affect anyone, including breast cancer patients. Common symptoms include sadness, hopelessness, and loss of interest in activities that were once enjoyable (anhedonia) for over two weeks.

Breast cancer patients may be at higher risk for depression due to the emotional and physical stress of the diagnosis and treatment and the potential impact on their relationships, work, and overall quality of life. Specific breast cancer treatments, such as chemotherapy and hormonal therapy, may also cause depression as a side effect.

Breast cancer patients need to be aware of the signs and symptoms of depression, such as persistent sadness, fatigue, difficulty sleeping, and changes in appetite or weight. They should notify their healthcare provider or a mental health professional promptly. If left untreated, depression can have serious consequences, including impaired functioning, decreased quality of life, and an increased risk of suicide.

Treatment options for depression in breast cancer patients may include psychotherapy, medication, or a combination. Cognitive-behavioral therapy (CBT) and other forms of talk therapy can help patients learn coping strategies to manage symptoms and improve their mood. Prescription medication with antidepressants also may help regulate mood and relieve symptoms.

In addition to these conventional treatments, patients may consider complementary therapies such as exercise, mindfulness meditation, and acupuncture. By addressing depression promptly and effectively, breast cancer patients can better cope with the challenges of the disease and its treatment. Remember, counselors, psychologists, psychiatrists, and other mental health professionals are part of the multidisciplinary team of a breast cancer patient during treatment and beyond.

Insomnia

Up to 70 percent of women newly diagnosed with breast cancer or who received recent treatment for breast cancer experience insomnia. It is double that of the general population. Insomnia exacerbates the other common symptoms of pain, fatigue, and depression that breast cancer patients experience—a combination that results in an overall decreased quality of life for women undergoing breast cancer therapy.

There are many reasons for sleep disturbances in a woman undergoing treatment for breast cancer. Cancer in and of itself is disruptive to our biological environment, both locally at the tumor site and distantly due to influencing hormones and steroid production. The pharmacological agents used to treat and help alleviate the side effects of treatment—that is, menopausal symptoms—can all cause insomnia. The adjustment to the numerous medical appointments and professional and personal obligations under a base of emotional and psychological distress contributes to poor sleep in a breast cancer patient.

In addition to using pharmacological agents with care (always consult with your doctor so as not to cause drug interactions with treating agents), cognitive behavioral therapy (CBT) and complementary alternative therapies such as yoga, meditation, and acupuncture help improve quality of life.

Chronic Fatigue

According to Berger et al., cancer-related fatigue (CRF) is defined as "a distressing, persistent, subjective sense of physical, emotional, and/or cognitive tiredness or exhaustion related to cancer or cancer treatment that is not proportional to recent activity and interferes with usual functioning."

Instruments to Assess Fatigue

- Breast Cancer Survivor Symptom Survey fatigue subscale
- Brief Fatigue Inventory
- European Organization for Research and Treatment of Cancer–Quality-of-Life Questionnaire (EORTC)-C30 fatigue subscale
- EORTC Quality of Life Module Measuring Cancer Related Fatigue (EORTC QLQ-FA12)
- Fatigue Symptom Inventory
- Memorial Symptoms Assessment Scale Short Form
- Piper Fatigue Scale revised
- Somatic and Psychological Health Report fatigue scale

Interventions to reduce fatigue among survivors of breast cancer post-treatment.

Non-Pharmacologic
- Counseling/education (delivered in person or remotely)
- Physical activity (maintaining recommended levels of activity, i.e., 150 minutes of moderate intensity activity/week, combining endurance and resistance training; beware of safety issues; personalize activity levels if needed; consider physical therapy and rehabilitation if needed)
- Other physical and mind–body interventions
- Yoga
- Massage therapy
- Acupuncture
- Music therapy
- Mindfulness meditation and relaxation
- Reiki
- Qigong
- Psychosocial interventions
- Psycho-educational therapies
- Cognitive-behavioral therapy
- Treatment for emotional distress
- Sleep hygiene

Pharmacologic
- Supplements (ginseng, vitamin D)

From: Long-Term Fatigue and Cognitive Disorders in Breast Cancer Survivors (Joly et al.)

BRAIN FOG

Brain fog, also known as chemo brain or cognitive dysfunction, is a common side effect of breast cancer treatment that can affect memory, concentration, and ability to process information. Some of the characteristic symptoms of brain fog are confusion, forgetfulness, and mental fatigue, and they can significantly impact the patient's quality of life even years after initial treatment.

The cause of brain fog is unknown. It is likely related to cancer treatment and other factors such as stress, anxiety, and depression. Chemotherapy, hormonal, and radiation therapy can cause inflammation, which may contribute to the development of brain fog.

Cognitive exercises, lifestyle changes, and medication are strategies to manage brain fog. Mental exercises, such as puzzles or memory games, can help improve memory and concentration. Practicing good sleep hygiene is an underrated but effective solution. A healthy diet and regular physical activity will help with brain fog, supporting overall brain health.

COMPLEMENTARY AND ALTERNATIVE MEDICINE (CAM)

Complementary and alternative medicine (CAM) refers to a range of medical practices and treatments that fall outside of conventional Western medicine. These therapies may be used alongside or in place of standard medical treatments for breast cancer.

Some examples of CAM therapies commonly used by breast cancer patients include acupuncture, massage therapy, yoga, and meditation. Other CAM treatments, such as dietary supplements, herbs, and homeopathic remedies, are also sometimes used.

While some patients may find CAM therapies helpful in managing symptoms or improving quality of life, approach these treatments with caution. Many CAM therapies have yet to be rigorously studied for their safety or effectiveness, and some may even be harmful or interfere with conventional medical treatments. Patients interested in using CAM therapies should discuss their options with their healthcare providers and seek out practitioners licensed and trained in their chosen therapy. Potential risks and interactions with conventional medical treatment is possible, and extra caution is necessary when considering using unproven or untested therapies.

In some cases, healthcare providers may recommend CAM therapies as part of a comprehensive treatment plan for breast cancer. For example, some studies have suggested that acupuncture may be effective in reducing chemotherapy-induced nausea and vomiting. At the same time, yoga and meditation may help reduce stress and anxiety.

Ultimately, the decision to use CAM therapies is personal, and patients should work closely with their healthcare providers to determine the best course of treatment for their individual needs and circumstances. By combining conventional medical treatments with evidence-based CAM therapies, patients may improve their quality of life and better manage breast cancer's physical and emotional challenges.

Acupuncture

Acupuncture is a traditional Chinese medical practice during which thin needles are inserted into specific parts of the body based on the Meridian system. It treats various conditions, including pain, nausea, anxiety, infertility, and depression.

In the context of breast cancer, acupuncture has been studied as a complementary therapy for managing treatment-related symptoms, such as pain, fatigue, and nausea. Several clinical trials have suggested that acupuncture may be effective in reducing chemotherapy-induced gastrointestinal symptoms, such as nausea and vomiting, and in improving the quality of life in breast cancer patients.

The mechanism by which acupuncture works is yet to be fully understood. It is known to promote the release of endorphins, which are natural painkillers that may stimulate the body's biological healing processes.

Acupuncture is a safe practice when performed by a licensed practitioner. However, it is not suitable for everyone. Pregnant women or people with certain medical conditions, such as bleeding disorders, should not undergo acupuncture treatment without consulting their healthcare provider first.

Keep in mind that acupuncture is a complementary therapy for breast cancer patients to help manage specific symptoms and improve quality of life. It is not a substitute for conventional medical treatments for breast cancer, such as surgery, chemotherapy, or radiation therapy.

Overall, patients interested in using acupuncture as a complementary therapy should discuss their options with their healthcare provider and seek a licensed practitioner with experience treating breast cancer patients. By working closely with their healthcare team and incorporating evidence-based complementary therapies into their overall treatment plan, breast cancer patients may achieve better outcomes and improved quality of life.

Vitamin D

Vitamin D is a hormone that plays an essential role in bone health, immune function, development, and cell growth, among others. It may have a protective effect against certain types of cancer, including breast cancer.

Low levels of vitamin D may be a risk factor for breast cancer. A higher risk of recurrence and poorer outcomes during treatment for breast cancer have also been associated with low levels of vitamin D. A meta-analysis by Chen et al. showed an inverse relationship between vitamin D levels and breast cancer risk. The scientific evidence regarding the relationship between vitamin D and breast cancer is still evolving. Continued research is needed for a better understanding of the mechanism and relationship.

A common source of vitamin D is from the skin after sunlight exposure. Foods in your diet, such as fatty fish, eggs, and fortified dairy products, are also good sources. Unfortunately, many people do not get enough vitamin D from their diet or sun exposure alone. For this reason, breast cancer patients are advised to take vitamin D supplements to help maintain optimal levels.

The recommended daily vitamin D intake varies depending on age, sex, and overall health status. Excessive intake of vitamin D supplements may cause elevated calcium levels, which may lead to gastrointestinal upset, bone pain, and kidney problems. Your healthcare provider should help in determining the appropriate levels.

MEDICAL AND IMAGING SURVEILLANCE

Women with a history of breast cancer have an increased risk of developing recurrent cancer in the treated breast, a new cancer in the treated breast, cancer in the opposite breast, and axillary or distant metastasis. Clinical and imaging follow-up is based on the stage of the cancer at diagnosis, disease progression, treatment protocols, and other factors unique to that patient. Most women today are treated with breast conservation therapy (BCT) with a lumpectomy and radiation therapy. In general, after the initial treatment of breast cancer, patients will have a clinical visit with the oncology team usually every six months for five years, then annually after.

Mammography is the standard imaging modality used for the surveillance of breast cancer after primary treatment. The frequency of surveillance imaging varies by institution. A diagnostic mammogram six months after the completion of radiation therapy, then annually or every six months for two years, is practiced at some institutions. Others may image every six months for up to five years. Annual screening breast MRIs in conjunction with mammograms may be performed for patients with genetic mutations, a strong family history, and elevated lifetime risk greater than 20 percent. Some doctors perform an annual MRI for younger patients, or patients whose cancer was mammographically occult and only seen on an MRI. According to an American Cancer Society (ACS) expert panel in 2007, a personal history of breast cancer alone does not justify overall screening of women who have undergone breast conservation therapy with an MRI. Other breast imaging modalities, such as ultrasound, positron emission tomography–computed tomography (PET/CT), and contrast mammography, are not routinely used except for a case-by-case basis and based on additional risk factors.

Patients who have had a bilateral mastectomy with or without breast reconstruction do not undergo routine imaging. Diagnostic imaging evaluation, typically starting with a mammogram and ultrasound, is performed when there are new or worrisome clinical or physical examination findings. Likewise, women with a unilateral mastectomy with or without reconstruction also do not undergo routine imaging of the postoperative breast but *will* undergo the usual annual screening mammogram of the unaffected breast.

Staging examinations with computed tomography (CT), bone scans, and PET/CT are performed routinely on a case-by-case basis only or if there are new symptoms suspicious for recurrent, new, or metastatic disease.

FEAR OF RECURRENCE

Fear of cancer recurrence is real! It is always in the back of a breast cancer survivor's mind, and it is worsened at the time of the annual mammogram and other imaging surveillance, so much so that there is a term for it—"scanxiety." Scanxiety is the emotion of fear, anxiety, and pseudo-symptoms that are triggered by routine or recommended tests for an ongoing chronic disease, usually cancer. For days, weeks, or even months before a test, some women experience anxiety, fear, and worry about worsening or recurrent disease. These emotions can lead to sleepless nights, headaches, abdominal pain, pain at the site of surgery—you name it! This may subside after a negative study or good news about favorable therapy response, only to return when it's time for testing again!

SIGNS OF BREAST CANCER RECURRENCE

There is a chance that breast cancer can recur in a period of up to thirty-two years, according to a Danish study published in 2022 (Pederson et al.). Recurrence is based on stage at diagnosis, size and extent of tumor, lymph node involvement receptor status (usually ER positive), and age (i.e., younger women). As much as one doesn't want to live in constant fear of cancer returning, there are some signs you should notify your doctor about, especially if they are new or worsening:

- Bone pain/fracture
- Shortness of breath (especially with daily activities and minimal exertion)
- Persistent cough
- Blurry vision
- Headaches
- Memory loss
- Unintentional weight loss
- Skin lesions especially at surgical site
- Early satiety and increase in size of abdomen
- Constipation or bloody stool

COMMUNITY AND SUPPORT GROUP RESOURCES

A breast cancer survivor should not and does not have to go at it alone. Support groups both online and offline are a tremendous resource. Support groups are a fantastic way to connect with other women who can relate to what you've been through and are going through. It is also a way to stay connected to experts and other resources available in your community. Life after cancer, in my opinion, is not a time to be a lone warrior.

You can create a free survivorship care plan through the University of Pennsylvania's OncoLife plan at oncolink.org.

MAIN TAKEAWAYS

Life after a breast cancer diagnosis is a journey filled with challenges, growth, and hope. It requires ongoing support and care. Surviving breast cancer is not only about overcoming the disease, but also about embracing a new normal and finding strength in the journey. Even when the physical battle against breast cancer is won, the emotional and psychological impact can linger. Self-care, both physically and emotionally, must be prioritized. While the fear of recurrence may linger, it is important to focus on living fully in the present moment and celebrating milestones. Surrounding yourself with a supportive network of loved ones and fellow survivors can provide invaluable encouragement and understanding. A breast cancer survivor is resilient, courageous, and deserving of a fulfilling life beyond cancer.

CHAPTER 12
LOVE YOUR BREASTS; LOVE YOURSELF

*You yourself, as much as anybody in the entire
universe, deserve your love and affection.*
—Buddha

YOUR PURPOSE, MISSION, MANDATE, DREAMS, and aspirations will impact your relationships, wealth, and legacy; it all hinges on good health. According to the World Health Organization (WHO), "Health is a state of complete physical, mental, and social well-being and merely the absence of disease."

The strong, beautiful, and courageous woman that you are, who takes care of her family, friends, co-workers, and everyone else, must also take care of herself. Like most of us on planet Earth these days, there's so much to do and not enough time. It feels like you need to make an appointment to meet up with yourself. Guess what? In this day and age, you do. Do you ever wonder how there never seems to be time for yourself, but somehow, you can always make time for others? The truth is it's because you have yet to make yourself a priority. It is essential to become self-aware of the implications of being at the bottom of the totem pole in your life! When your self-care, mind, and body become your top priority, the benefits ripple to your loved ones, workplace, projects, and community. It's a win-win.

Easier said than done, right? Nevertheless, it would be best if you committed to stop being visibly invisible in your life. It is especially true for Black women, where research studies have shown that photos of Black women go unrecognized the most, and their voices are least likely to be correctly attributed during a group discussion (see Sesko; Fryberg; and Purdie-Vaughns). Black women have been dehumanized for so long in modern society that we subconsciously play along with the narrative projected on us to be visibly invisible, present but unseen, and heard but discounted. Nobody sees you, and eventually, you no longer see yourself. Our self-image, self-worth, and authentic self must be fiercely empowered and protected. Practicing self-love through the lens of self-compassion, kindness to self, and mindfulness is essential for living a life of purpose with conscious choice and on your terms. And that begins with taking charge of your health.

In my practice as a breast radiologist, I'm often the first day and first moment in the rest of the life of a breast cancer patient. Understandably, most women think they have breast cancer when they feel a lump, need additional imaging after a screening mammogram, or need a biopsy. Unfortunately, in the small percentage that gets the phone call that confirms a cancer diagnosis, the week-long holding of their breath is released as a heavy, overwhelming sigh when the news is finally delivered. It's a sigh intermingled with shock, denial, confusion, and fear. The fear that caused the anxiety, delay, or avoidance of getting a mammogram in the first place is now confirmed and justified. When cancer appears to be in an early stage, I encourage my patients with positive survival outcomes and statistics. When the tumor is large and rapidly progressing, I still encourage my patients with the advancements made in treatment, affirming that there is always hope regardless of the cancer size or grade stage.

Most patients have an excellent prognosis from breast cancer when detected and treated early. Therefore, you must courageously commit to your health and wellness by participating in preventative screening exams. They stack the odds in your favor, which is excellent. It is especially the case with screening mammograms when one considers that breast cancer is the number-one cancer diagnosis in women and the highest cause of cancer deaths in women. In the United States, Black women fare worse than their counterparts, with a higher incidence of aggressive breast cancer subtypes and a higher mortality rate when compared with other groups of women. No matter who you are, where you live, or where you come from, when you feel a lump, new changes, or other concerning findings in your breast, please seek prompt medical evaluation and practice the recommended preventative health screening guidelines appropriate for your age. Don't let fear or disempowering beliefs stop you.

Often what holds us back is the fear of pain. As humans, we are motivated primarily by pain or pleasure. We move toward pleasure and do everything to remove pain. Medical preventative screenings in our minds are not pleasurable. In the case of "squishy" mammograms, the thought of pain comes to mind. So, it's not pleasant and perceived as a source of discomfort by some. In that case, it is understandably an examination process that many women would like to avoid. It makes sense—except we're talking about a medical examination that may save your life. Instead of avoiding the pain of the screening test, try and think about it differently. The disease we're trying to detect early, such as cancer, is typically painless and asymptomatic in its early stages, but it will eventually cause pain at advanced stages because of limited treatment options. Thus, catching it early means *less* pain in the long run. Reframing it this way helps to overcome the negative thoughts and ideas around a test scientifically proven to save lives. It is like exercising and eating healthily. It doesn't feel pleasurable and may even be downright painful in the beginning—until we start feeling, seeing, and reaping the benefits, which bring us the pleasure of improved self-esteem, self-confidence, zest, and vitality.

Learning to love yourself deeply and compassionately starts with you, and your mindset is everything. A mindset shift to one that is empowering is the most lasting change you can make, with the most significant ripple effect in every area of your life. Changing your mindset around preventive healthcare and beneficial activities that may not be pleasurable initially or that you perceive will cause you pain pays massive dividends. Limiting beliefs, such as cancer phobia and fatalistic and flawed health belief models, must be challenged. Health is crucial in pursuing happiness with a meaningful and fulfilled lifestyle. Dedication and commitment to your health are part of the journey to becoming a more authentic, higher, and better version of yourself. It is one of the manifestations of self-love. Jim Rohn puts it perfectly: "Take care of your body. It's the only place you have to live."

We take it for granted, but taking care of oneself is an opportunity for and at life. Stand up for your life today! It is easier said than done, right? Many triggers, self-sabotaging, and self-handicapping beliefs and behaviors limit you in seeking a healthier you and the life you desire—for example, fear and limiting or disempowering attitudes and beliefs, such as fatalistic health beliefs.

FEAR

If you're afraid of the healthcare system or of going to the doctor's office, you must tease out why you're so scared. There are many reasons for fear: fear of receiving bad news, fear of cancer, fear of being disrespected or mistreated, fear of death, etc. It is best to overcome this fear because fear is not a cure or an empowering strategy. Being afraid and choosing denial doesn't change the facts. Courage, despite fear, is a better strategy because it will get you to the other side of fear, where hope, freedom, and healing reside.

By acting, you empower yourself, step over your fears, and give feedback to your subconscious mind that "I have the power to handle anything that comes my way. I choose to be proactive, and if something is wrong, it will be detected on time, thereby allowing me to take advantage of early detection and the treatments available to me." You must delve into your subconscious mind and get to the root of your fears. As humans, we are born with two fears: fear of falling and fear of loud noises. That's it. So where do the *other* fears come from? They are learned behaviors based on personal life experiences, beliefs, thought patterns, culture, environment, and society.

LIMITING OR DISEMPOWERING ATTITUDES AND BELIEFS

We often don't know when limiting beliefs and false ideologies creep into and take root in our subconscious minds. If you do a bit of reflection, you may discover that your resistance to health-seeking behaviors may be rooted in a negative experience with the healthcare system during childhood. Seemingly harmless statements from family and friends who don't like doctors/healthcare systems may also impact your belief system and the utility of health-seeking behaviors. You may have repeatedly heard statements like "No news is good news," "If it ain't broke, don't fix it," or "If I go to the doctor, they're going to find something wrong with me." In no time, this soon becomes your belief too!

Due to a complex combination of factors—such as socioeconomic status, health disparities, and genetics—the Black community tends to have poorer outcomes for certain major diseases compared to some other groups. So, when people in your environment make statements like "No news is good news" or "If I go to a doctor, they'll tell me something is wrong," please keep in mind the statistically worse outcomes of certain diseases in these communities. Limiting or disempowering beliefs and statements, as well as fatalistic health belief models, contribute to the high rates of premature death in our communities from often curable and medically manageable diseases. You should no longer buy into or be passive about such narratives. Instead, engage in empowered actions to prevent ending up as a negative statistic. As a community, we must work on modifying attitudes and beliefs that do not empower but ultimately have detrimental outcomes and effects.

Committing to mindset change and then to a lifestyle change can revolutionize your life: it can open up pathways to self-discovery, self-awareness, and self-compassion and help you answer powerful questions, such as: What's your why? How do you design the extraordinary, harmonious, and fulfilling life you desire? What does that life look like? How do you bring that life into existence? How do you set and achieve goals based on your North Star? Is your rudder facing the right direction? How do you become the embodiment of that which you seek and value? Once you find those answers, you must commit to change—and then you must *act* to achieve the transformation you want. How? It begins with self-love.

L.O.V.E. CONQUERS ALL

I am the master of my fate. I am the captain of my soul.
—William Ernest Henley, "Invictus"

All we need is love. It sounds cliché, but all we need is love, which truly does conquer all. We've discussed breast health and the importance of living a healthy and empowered life. So, what's love got to do with it? Everything!

"You shall love your God with all your heart and love your neighbor as you love yourself." As a Nigerian raised with Judeo-Christian values, this New Testament bible verse from Mark chapter 10 was drilled into me repeatedly at home, school, church, and everywhere I went as a child.

I was well into my thirties before I realized I only practiced two out of the three directives of this bible verse and was neglectful of the crucial third—as were most people I knew! Loving God and my neighbor, I had that down pat in my way. However, through parental, cultural, and societal norms, intentionally and unconsciously, any portrayed or perceived acts of self-love for me were labeled as selfish, self-serving, unworthy, unbecoming, and forbidden territory.

The absence and suppression of the third component of Mark chapter 10—to love myself—persisted until I asked myself the paradigm-shifting question, "Who am I and why am I here?" This question emerged into my consciousness during the turbulent transition from medical student to intern, with its hectic work schedules, increased responsibilities, emotional roller coasters, and a heavy dose of self-doubt. This powerful question blindsided me and brought me to a grinding halt, spiritually, emotionally, and mentally. I became confused, depressed, and dumbfounded that I could not respond coherently to those eight words. I did not know "my why." I had been cruising on planet Earth for thirty years, came from a large family, grew up in a bustling city, served five years in the United States Navy with an honorable discharge, graduated from college, was well-traveled, married, attended Medical School, graduated in the top 5 percent of my class, and was headed to the ivory tower for a radiology residency. I had accomplished many things and was at the "top of my game." Yet, I did not have a well-articulated understanding of who I was, my why, or who was in the driver's seat of my life. At age thirty, I became aware, for the first time, that I lacked self-awareness. I did not know myself, and I most certainly wasn't a practitioner of authentic self-love.

This pivotal moment in my life was the beginning of my personal development journey in self-discovery, self-awareness, self-mastery, and self-expression. It has been transformative thus far, and I'm only scratching the surface. To date, my most profound and most reassuring affirmation from a culmination of my life experiences, mentorships, and moments of reflection is that "I deeply and compassionately love myself just the way that I am." My desire for you is that you feel and experience the same.

LOVE YOUR BREASTS: LOVE YOURSELF

Number one in your life's blueprint should be a deep belief in your own dignity, your worth, and your own somebodiness. Do not allow anybody to make you feel that you're nobody. Always feel that you count. Always feel that you have worth, and always feel that your life has ultimate significance.
—Martin Luther King Jr.

As a woman, you may feel visibly invisible, discounted, or told that you are undesirable and at the "bottom of the totem pole," as many of us have either heard or been made to feel. In a continual battle to prove your self-worth, you prioritize others before yourself by getting busy with everything and everyone else but you. You soon forget you are also worthy of love, recognition, and value. You've maneuvered the world under the radar and out of the way for so long that you've become invisible to yourself. As the beautiful warrior and shining light you are, you must push back on narratives, beliefs, stereotypes, and ideologies that don't enrich or serve you. They are disempowering, limiting, harmful, unfair, and untrue. Let your light shine by loving yourself in all your magnificence and glory. You are somebody, and you are enough.

I encourage you to become an intentional self-advocate for yourself and your health. Value your value! Prioritize yourself. Fear, limiting beliefs, and the negative attitudes projected by others should not stop you from taking care of and speaking up for number one—you. Your body provides empowerment, enrichment, enjoyment, and freedom. As the saying goes, "Health is wealth." Therefore, it is essential to be proactive and informed about your breast and overall health. We have not been given a spirit of fear, but of love, power, and a sound mind.

Love your breasts—no matter the narrative around them, no matter their shape or size. Take the time to acknowledge and get to know them and yourself, from understanding what they can do to becoming familiar with the changes that can occur. Knowledge is power! Educate yourself so you can empower yourself, and advocate for your health. This is what I want for you. This is why I wrote this book: so you have the knowledge and encouragement to help you love your breasts, love yourself just the way you are, and act when necessary.

Self-love is not selfish; you cannot truly love another until you know how to love yourself.
—Unknown

MAIN TAKEAWAYS

The greatest act of self-love is embracing and accepting oneself fully. It involves practicing self-compassion, treating oneself with kindness and understanding, and letting go of self-criticism and judgment. Self-love is recognizing your worth, honoring your needs, and setting healthy boundaries. It involves prioritizing your physical, emotional, and mental well-being above external expectations or societal pressures. By nurturing a positive and supportive relationship with yourself, you cultivate a deep sense of inner peace. This foundation of self-love enables you to prioritize your well-being and pursue your passions and goals with confidence and authenticity. Self-love is committing to your growth, happiness, and fulfillment, knowing that you deserve love, acceptance, and joy in every aspect of your life.

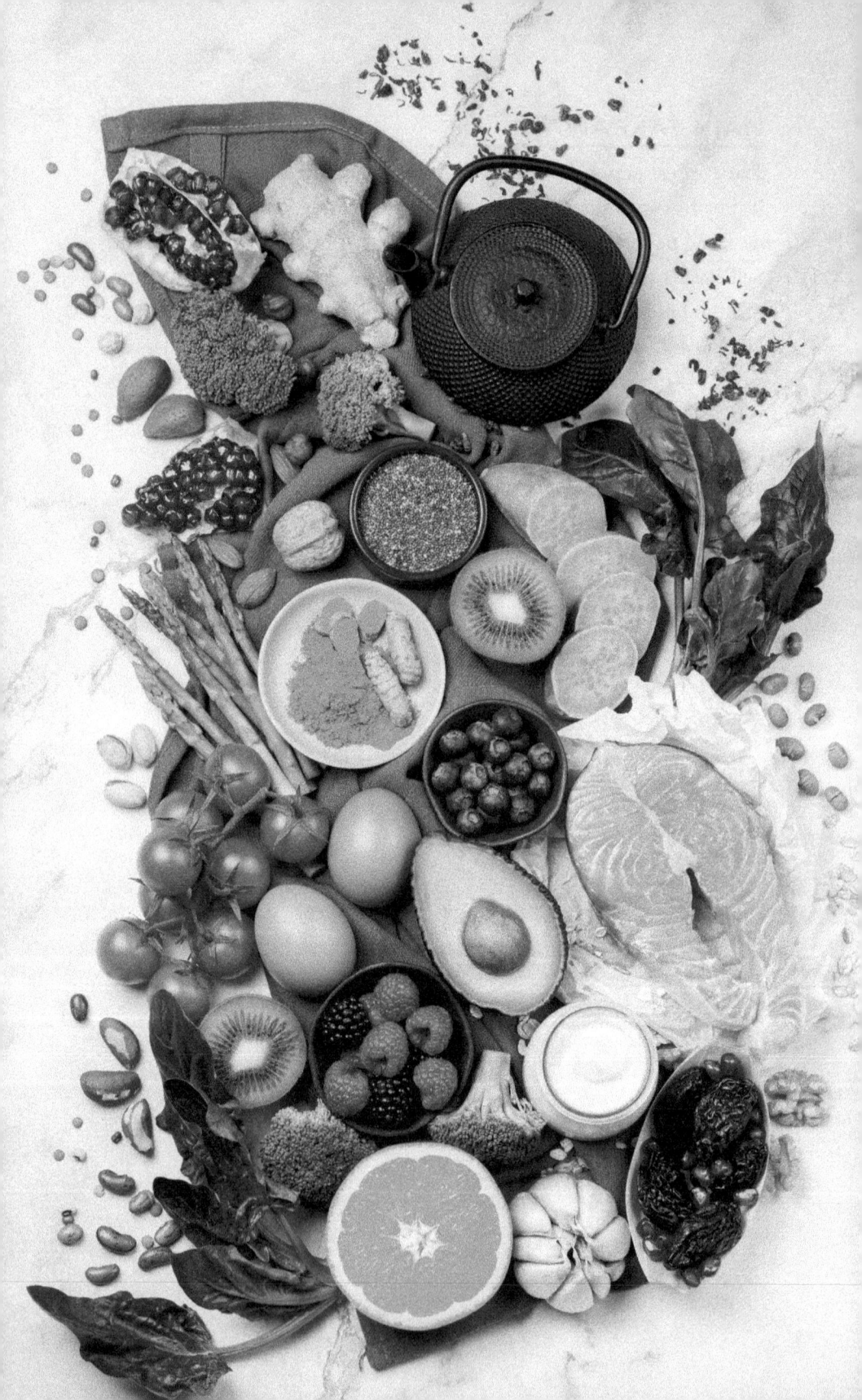

SECTION 4
DIET FOR BREAST HEALTH

Love Your Breasts by Eating Well

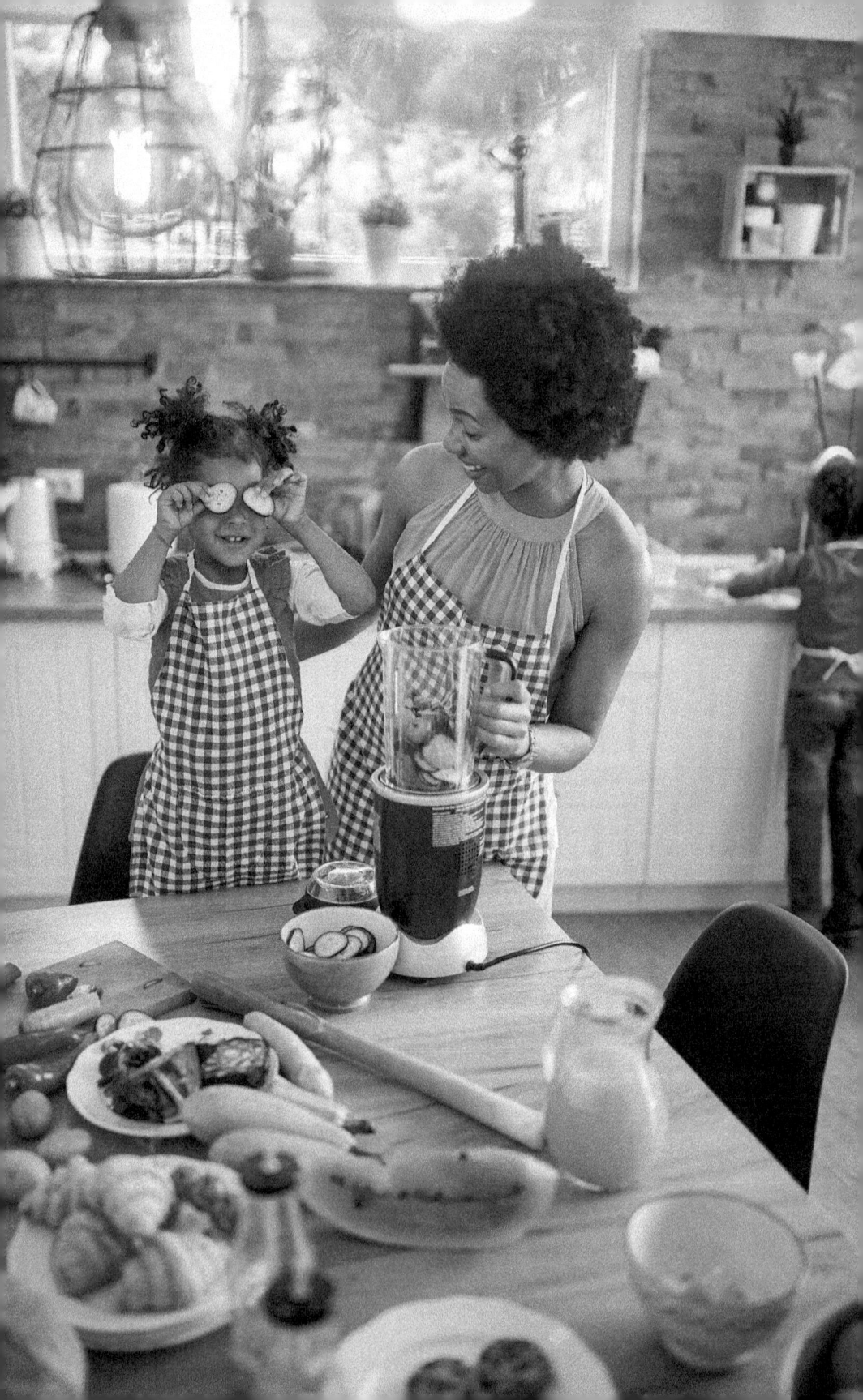

YOUR BREAST HEALTH and your overall health, for that matter, is influenced by your genetics and your environment. We cannot modify out genetics, but we have some control over our environment, including lifestyle choices like diet.

Through our diet, we provide our bodies with the nutrients to help ensure our cells, organs, and systems have everything they need to function properly and fight off illness.

When it comes to our breasts, researchers have identified dietary habits that help to promote breast health, as well as types of foods that provide us with nutrients and other components that go the extra mile to support our immune system.

The dietary pattern that is generally best for supporting breast health is one that is low in saturated fat, high in fruits and vegetables, and rich in whole grains and lean protein.

In this recipe book, we have created delicious meals, snacks, and drinks that we hope will inspire you to eat nutrient-rich foods that will support your breast health. We encourage you to choose a few recipes and start integrating them into your diet. After a few weeks, ask yourself how you feel.

We are confident that these recipes will help you feel energized, healthy, and satisfied so you can turn over a new leaf and make a conscious effort to make decisions that support your breast health.

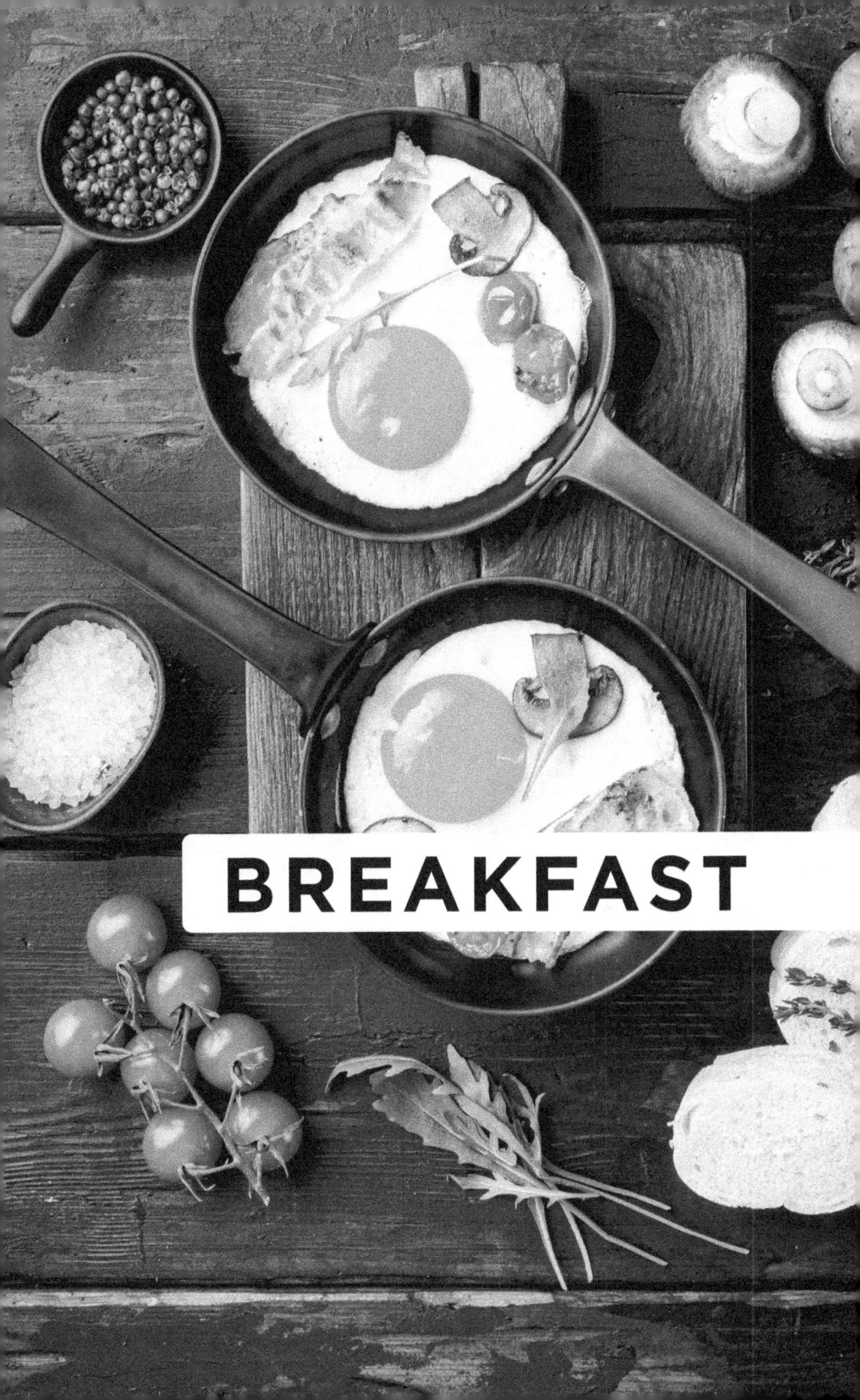

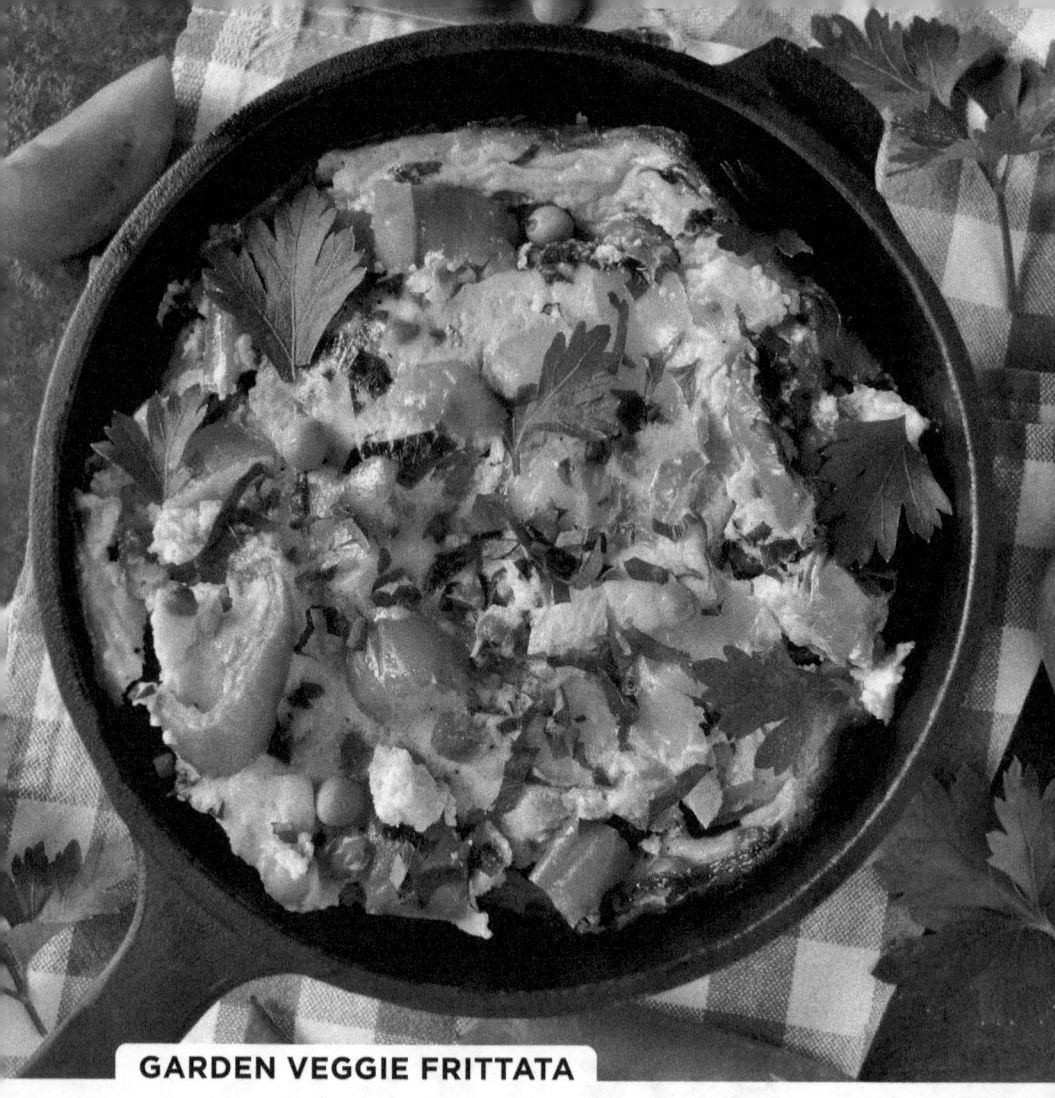

GARDEN VEGGIE FRITTATA

Prep time: 10 minutes   Cook time: 20 minutes   Servings: 4

THE WHOLE FAMILY WILL ENJOY this frittata recipe. It includes cruciferous and allium vegetables, which are high in vitamins, minerals, and phytochemicals that support breast health in two ways: they help strengthen your immune system and scavenge free radicals that could damage breast cells. Rather than using butter, this recipe uses olive oil, which is rich in omega-3 fatty acids, which research has shown helps to inhibit the growth of breast tumors.

Ingredients

- 3 whole eggs
- 4 egg whites
- ¼ cup mozzarella cheese, shredded
- 1 cup broccoli florets
- ¼ cup red onion, sliced
- ½ cup tomatoes, diced
- ¼ cup bell pepper, diced
- 1 tbsp fresh basil
- 1 tbsp extra virgin olive oil
- Salt and pepper to taste

Directions

1. Preheat the oven to 220°C.
2. In a medium bowl, whisk together the eggs, mozzarella, basil, salt, and pepper.
3. On the stovetop, heat olive oil in a cast iron or oven-safe pan.
4. Add vegetables to the pan and sauté for about 3 minutes until the broccoli florets soften slightly. Don't worry if they are still crisp! The vegetables will soften up in the oven.
5. Pour the egg mixture over the vegetables and place in the oven.
6. Bake the mixture, uncovered, for about 20 minutes, or until the center of the frittata is cooked through.

Nutrition Facts

- Calories: 117 (5.6%)
- Total Fat: 7.3 g (9%)
- Saturated Fat: 1.7 g (9%)
- Carbohydrates: 4.2 g (2%)
- Dietary Fiber: 2.2 g (4g)
- Protein: 9.3 g

QUICK TIP

You can switch out the vegetables in this recipe for almost any vegetables you have in the fridge. Spinach, asparagus, and mushrooms make great additions and contribute antioxidants and fiber to the mix.

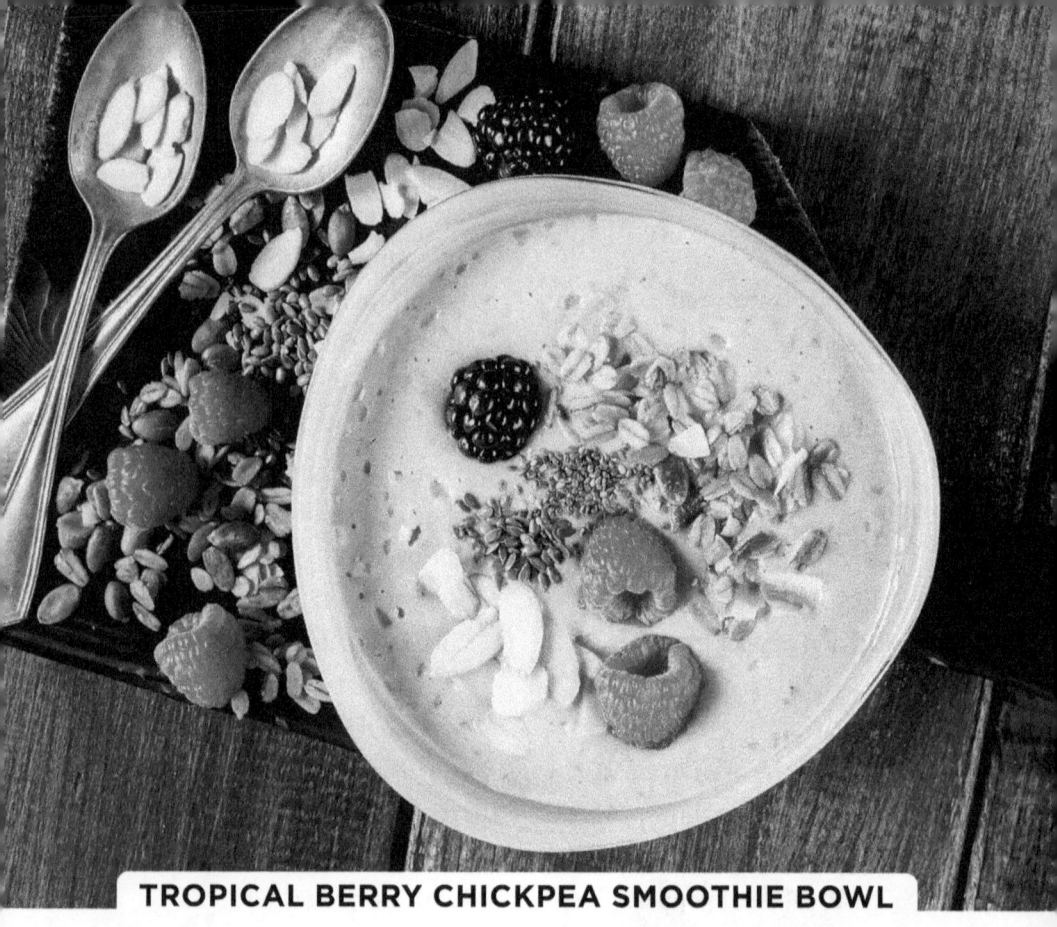

TROPICAL BERRY CHICKPEA SMOOTHIE BOWL

Prep time: 5 minutes   Cook time: 0 minutes   Servings: 1

DON'T THINK A SMOOTHIE WILL SUFFICE for breakfast? This chickpea smoothie bowl will surely change your mind. In fact, this energy-packed smoothie bowl is perfect if you have a busy day ahead because it will keep you energized and satisfied. This smoothie bowl alone will deliver almost 90 percent of your recommended daily intake of fiber.

    The chickpeas add fiber and protein, but the fruit gives it a delicious tropical twist. A couple of "hidden" ingredients, like the avocado and maca powder, elevate the anti-inflammatory properties of the smoothie bowl to support breast health and overall health. Top it all off with chia seeds, fresh berries, nuts, and oats, and you've got a satisfying breakfast that tastes like dessert!

BREAKFAST

Ingredients

- 1 cup mixed frozen berries (blueberries, blackberries, strawberries, and raspberries)
- ½ frozen banana
- ¼ cup canned chickpeas, rinsed
- ¼ avocado
- ½ orange, peeled
- 1 tsp maca powder (optional)
- ¾ cup unsweetened almond milk, or vegetable milk of your choice
- ¼ cup granola
- 1 tbsp crushed almonds (or nuts of your choice)
- ¼ cup fresh berries

Directions

1. Place all ingredients, except granola, almonds, and fresh berries, into a blender.
2. Blend until smooth.
3. Pour into a bowl and top with granola, almonds, and fresh berries.

Nutrition Facts

- Calories: 662 (33%)
- Total Fat: 38.1 g (49%)
- Saturated Fat: 5.7 g (28%)
- Carbohydrates: 118.7 g (43%)
- Dietary Fiber: 25.1 g (109%)
- Protein: 21.3 g

QUICK TIP

There is no "right way" to make a smoothie bowl. Adding your favorite spices and nutrient-packed toppings is a great way to make this part of your weekly meal plan. Adding cinnamon to the smoothie will make it spicier, while adding mint will give it a fresher taste. Feel free to experiment, and you'll soon see why smoothie bowls are so popular!

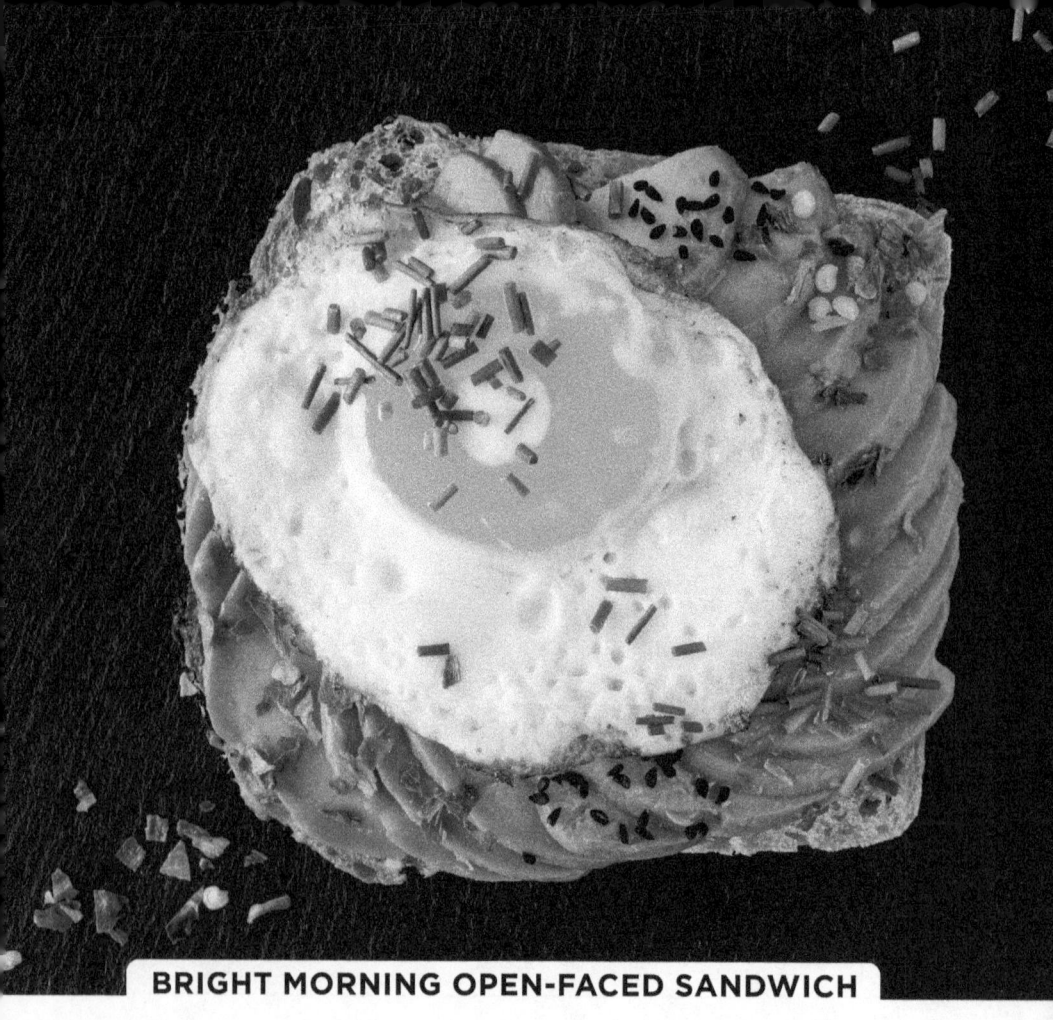

BRIGHT MORNING OPEN-FACED SANDWICH

Prep time: 5 minutes   Cook time: 5 minutes   Servings: 2

YES! YOU, TOO, CAN MAKE A BREAKFAST SANDWICH as bright, beautiful, and appetizing as this one. This recipe takes basic ingredients to make a filling, no-fork-needed breakfast you can enjoy at leisure or take with you on the go. The whole-wheat bread delivers filling fiber that will support heart health while also helping to balance your hormones. The avocado and egg yolks deliver healthy fats to help reduce inflammation, the egg whites provide complete proteins to keep you full and well-nourished, and the fresh spinach ensures you're getting your daily dose of antioxidants. Enjoy this recipe for breakfast or anytime of day!

Ingredients

- 2 slices of whole-wheat bread
- ½ avocado
- ½ tsp fresh lemon juice
- 1 tsp onion flakes
- 1 cup baby spinach
- 1 tsp olive oil
- 2 eggs
- Salt and pepper to taste
- Red pepper flakes (optional)
- Black sesame seeds and fresh fennel seeds for topping (optional)

Directions

1. Place slices of bread in toaster oven.
2. Scoop out avocado into a small bowl and mix in lemon juice and onion flakes. Mix until smooth and blended. Set aside.
3. Pour olive oil into a frying pan and heat to medium-low.
4. Add eggs to the frying pan and cook to your liking.
5. Spread avocado onto each slice of toast, divide spinach evenly between the pieces of toast, and place one egg on each one.
6. Sprinkle with salt and pepper to taste, and add pepper flakes, black sesame, and fennel, if desired.

Nutrition Facts

- Calories: 261 (13.1%)
- Total Fat: 12.6 g (22%)
- Saturated Fat: 3 g (20%)
- Carbohydrates: 15.3 g (17.5%)
- Dietary Fiber: 4 g (20%)
- Protein: 10.2 g

QUICK TIP

Has your doctor suggested that you keep an eye on your cholesterol levels? Cut out most of the cholesterol by getting rid of the egg yolk and using egg whites. Since it won't be as filling this way, feel free to double it up and have both pieces of toast for yourself.

Are you worried one slice of toast won't keep you satisfied for the busy day you have ahead? Accompany this open-faced toast with a cup of your favorite fruit or a smoothie for a more filling, energy-fuelled breakfast.

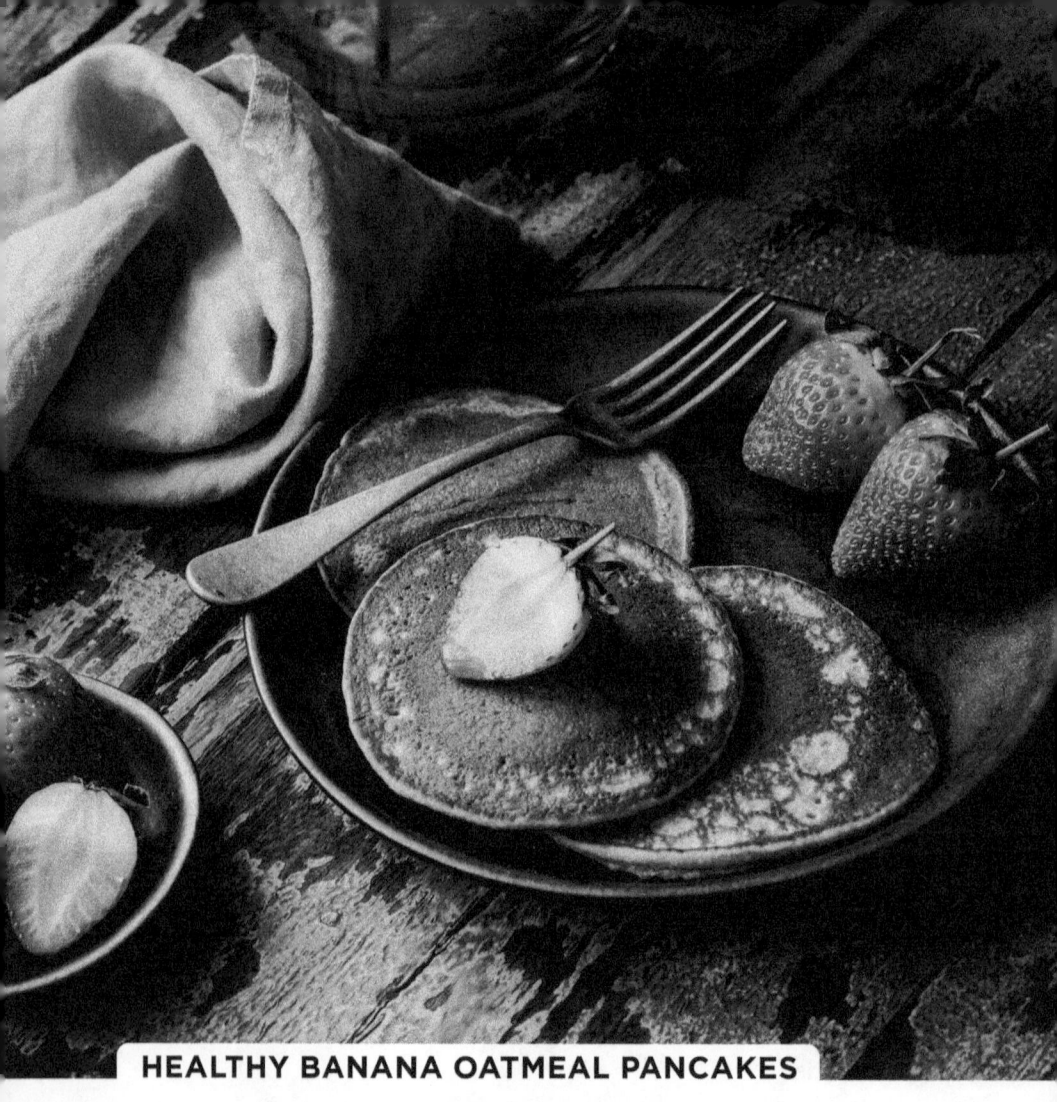

HEALTHY BANANA OATMEAL PANCAKES

Prep time: 5 minutes   Cook time: 10 minutes   Servings: 3

BOXED PANCAKE MIX IS EASY and pretty darn yummy, but most mixes contain refined flours, which strip away most of the fiber from the grain, as well as added sugars that, when consumed regularly, can cause inflammation. This pancake recipe is made with oatmeal, sweetened with banana, and contains nutrient-packed "superfoods" that support breast health with their anti-inflammatory and anti-oxidant components. Even the youngest ones in your family will love this recipe!

Ingredients

- 2 ripe bananas
- 2 eggs
- 1 cup rolled oats
- 1 tsp vanilla
- ½ tsp cinnamon
- 1 tbsp chia
- 1 tsp vegetable oil (for cooking)
- 2 tbsp honey (for topping)

Directions

1. Peel the bananas and place them in a medium bowl.
2. Mash the bananas with a fork until smooth.
3. Add the eggs and mix until blended. Mix in the rest of the ingredients (except for the oil).
4. In a large pan, heat up the oil on medium-low heat.
5. Pour pancake mix to make small pancakes (about 6–7 cm in diameter).
6. Wait for 1–2 minutes or until golden brown, and flip. When cooked through, remove from heat.
7. Serve with a drizzle of honey.

Nutrition Facts

- Calories: 301 (15%)
- Total Fat: 9.4 g (12%)
- Saturated Fat: 1.9 g (10%)
- Carbohydrates: 46.9 g (17%)
- Dietary Fiber: 8.3 g (29%)
- Protein: 9.7 g

QUICK TIP

Want to add some more protein and cut out the need for honey? Try topping your pancakes with low-fat, sugar-free yogurt or with your favorite nut butter. These alternatives will add flavor and protein to your breakfast.

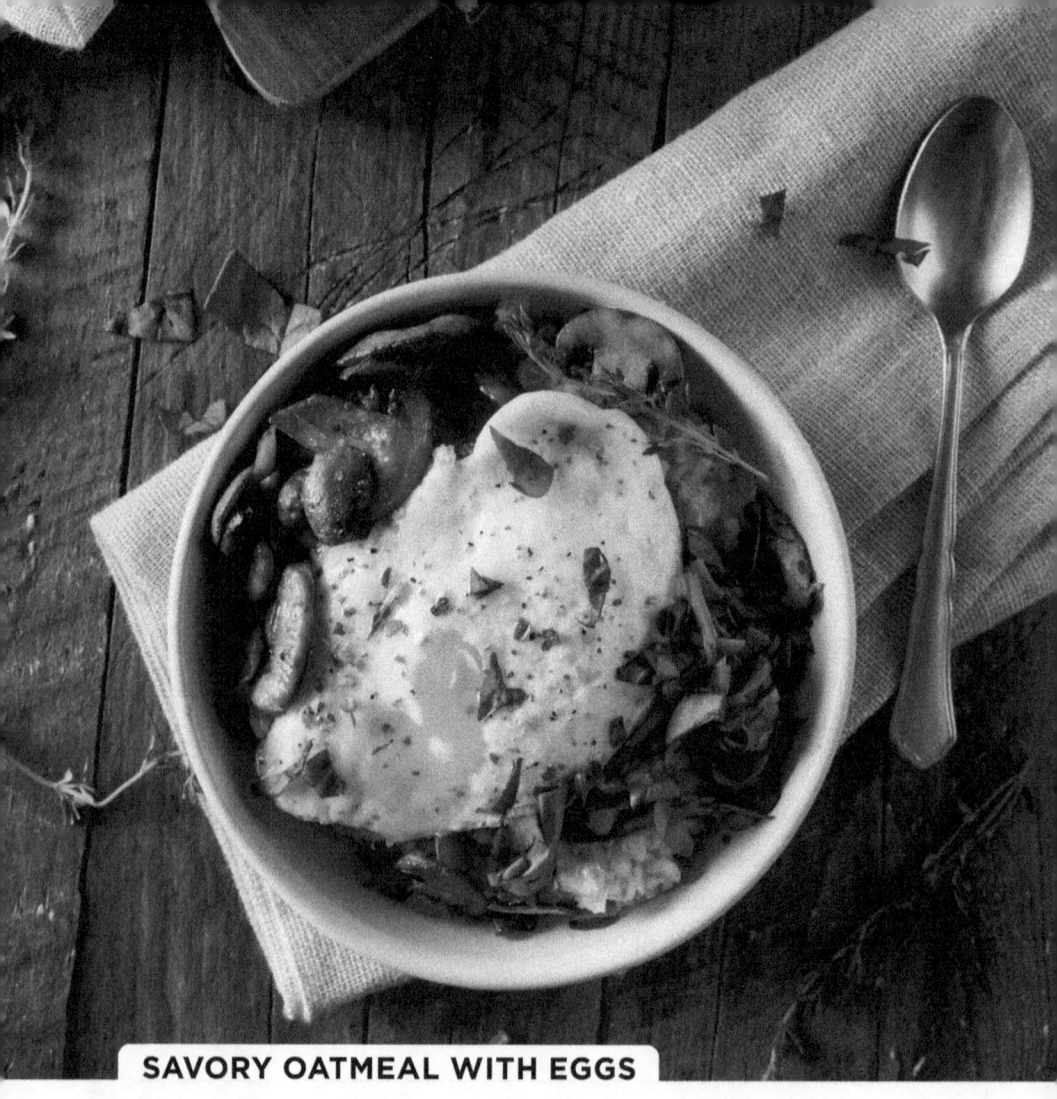

SAVORY OATMEAL WITH EGGS

Prep time: 5 minutes   Cook time: 10 minutes   Servings: 1

IF YOU'VE NEVER MADE SAVORY OATMEAL before, you don't know what you're missing. Adding an egg to your oatmeal makes it a more complete meal by providing your body with fats and protein in addition to whole-grain carbohydrates to fuel your day and provide you with balanced nutrition to support breast and full body health. Pair this hearty breakfast with a cup of your favorite berries for an antioxidant boost.

BREAKFAST

Ingredients

- 3/4 cup quick-cooking rolled oats
- 1 large egg
- 1 tbsp fresh scallions, sliced
- ½ tsp salt
- Cooking spray or ½ tsp olive oil
- ½ tsp freshly ground pepper
- Black sesame seeds and green onions or more scallions for garnishing (optional)
- Hot sauce (optional)

Nutrition Facts

- Calories: 326 (16.3%)
- Total Fat: 11.3 g (15%)
- Saturated Fat: 2.6 g (13%)
- Carbohydrates: 42.4 g (15%)
- Dietary Fiber: 6.4 g (23%)
- Protein: 14.5 g

Directions

1. In a small saucepan bring 1 cup water to boil.
2. Add the rolled oats and scallions with salt and pepper. Reduce to a simmer and cook until tender. Spray a small pan with cooking spray or pour in olive oil, then heat on medium low. Cook the egg to your liking.
3. Pour the oatmeal in a bowl, and carefully place egg on top.
4. Garnish with black sesame seeds and more scallions, if desired.

QUICK TIP

For a one-pot breakfast, you can break the egg into the oatmeal and mix it in as you cook it. The egg makes the oatmeal fluffier and almost buttery when you cook them together.

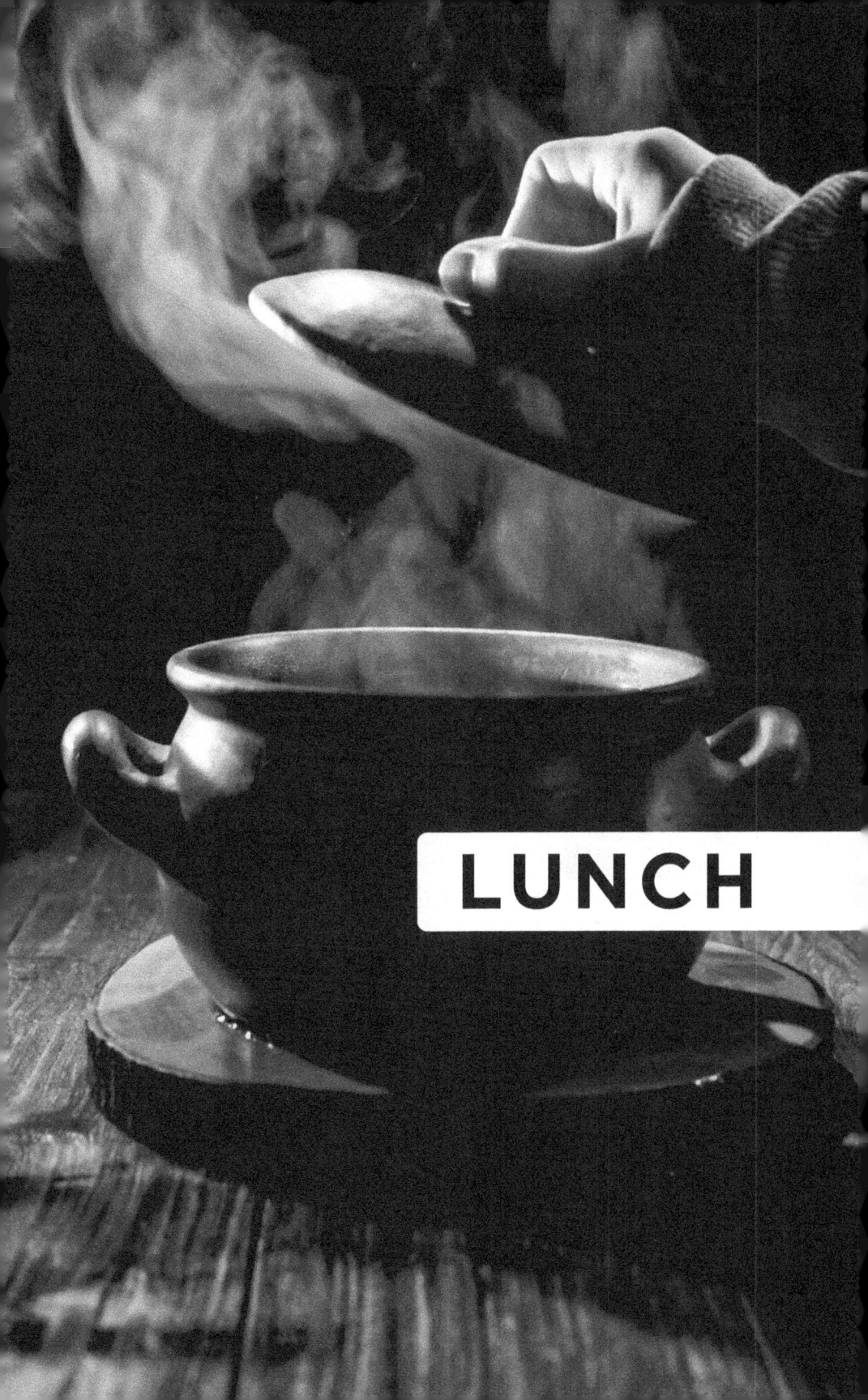

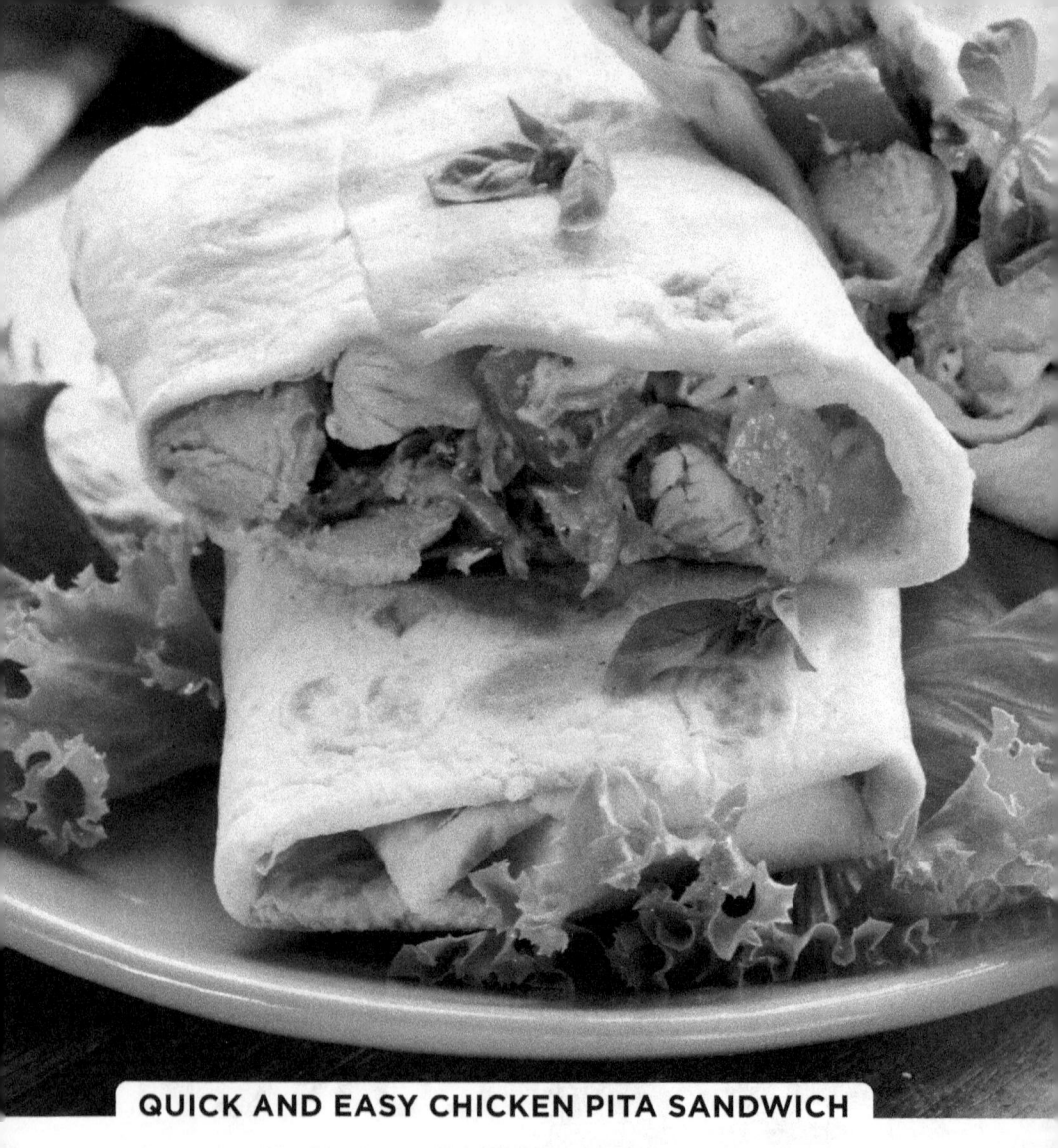

QUICK AND EASY CHICKEN PITA SANDWICH

Prep time: 15 minutes   Cook time: 0 minutes   Servings: 2

DO YOU NEED AN EASY-TO-MAKE LUNCH that is filling and nutritious? This chicken pita sandwich will soon become a regular go-to meal for you. The fiber-rich pita and vegetables may help to balance hormones that influence the appearance and development of hormone-dependent cancers, like some breast cancers. The chicken and fat-free Greek yogurt make this sandwich filling, while the fresh herbs and lime juice make it fresh and flavorful.

Ingredients

Filling
- 4 whole-wheat pita pocket halves
- ¼ rotisserie chicken or 2 leftover chicken breasts, shredded
- 1 cup lettuce, shredded
- ½ cucumber, sliced
- 2 tomatoes, sliced

Cucumber sauce
- ½ cup plain Greek yogurt
- ¼ cup cucumber, shredded
- 1 tbsp red onion, finely chopped
- 1 tsp parsley, minced
- 1 tbsp lime juice
- Dash garlic salt (or regular salt)
- Pepper to taste

Directions

1. In a small bowl, place the ingredients for the cucumber sauce and whisk together.
2. Using a butter knife, generously spread the sauce on the inside of the pita pockets.
3. In another bowl, toss together the filling ingredients.
4. Fill the pita pockets until stuffed to the brim.

Nutrition Facts

- Calories: 423 (21.2%)
- Total fat: 4.5 g (6%)
- Saturated fat: 1.6 g (8%)
- Total carbohydrates: 49.1 g (18%)
- Dietary Fiber: 2.9 g (10%)
- Protein: 42.2 g

QUICK TIP

If you don't have pita bread, you can use tortillas instead to make a wrap. Choose whole-wheat tortillas, when possible, to increase your fiber intake.

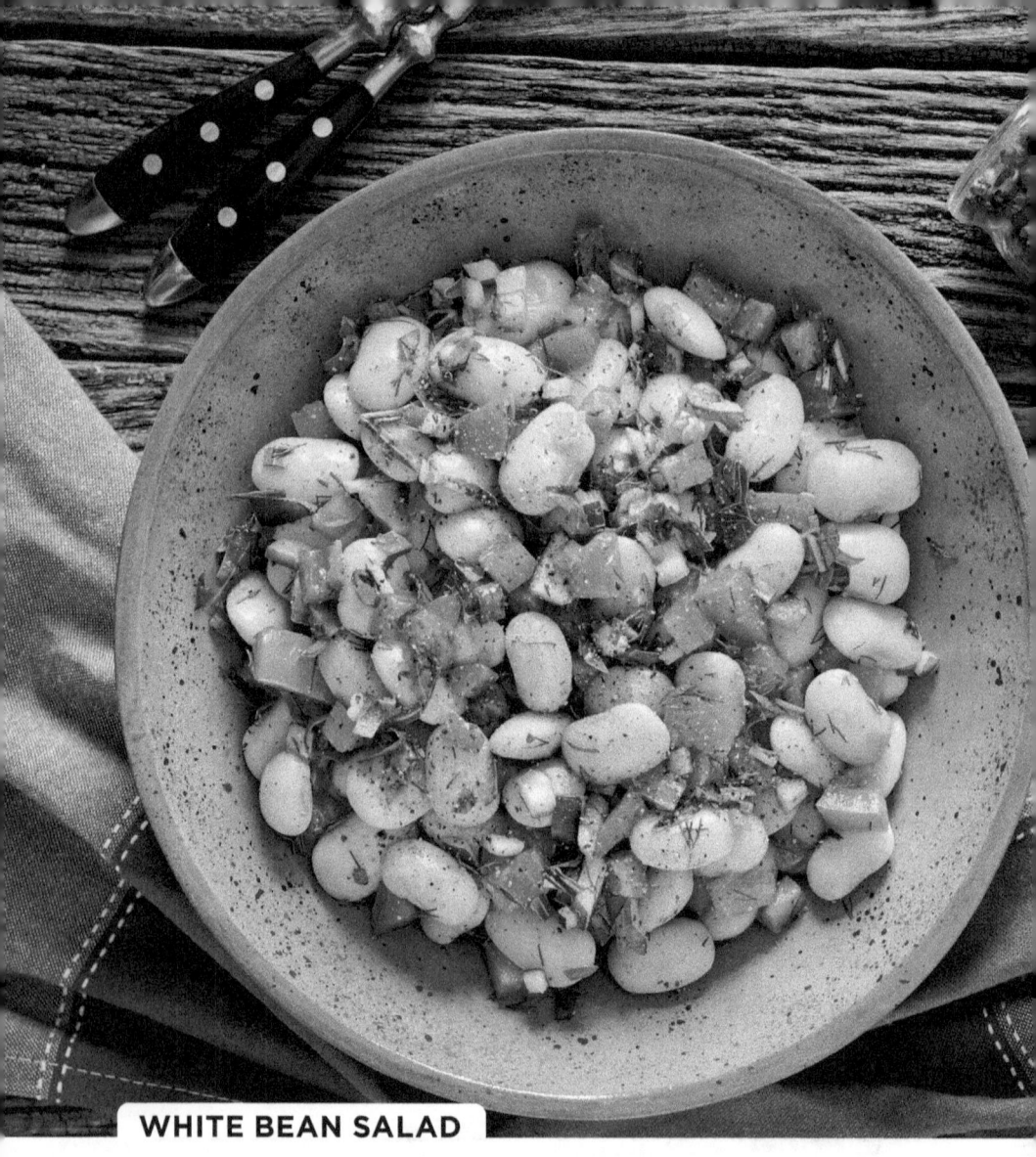

WHITE BEAN SALAD

Prep time: 20 minutes   Cook time: 0 minutes   Servings: 2

THIS SALAD IS A GREAT PLANT-BASED MEAL option for #MeatlessMondays or as a side for any dish. The white beans provide a meat-like texture and plenty of fiber to keep you satisfied. All of the ingredients deliver different kinds of antioxidants to help scavenge cancer-causing free radicals, including carotenoids from the bell pepper and tomatoes, flavonoids from the cilantro, organo-sulfides from the purple onion and shallots, and isoflavones from the white beans.

Ingredients

Salad

- 1 can white cannellini beans, drained and rinsed (or 1 ½ cup cooked white beans)
- 1 large tomato, chopped
- ¼ cup cilantro, chopped
- ½ purple onion, chopped
- 1 bell pepper, chopped

Dressing

- 2 tbsp olive oil
- 2 tbsp lime juice
- ½ shallot, minced
- 1 tsp honey
- Salt and pepper to taste

Directions

1. In a medium bowl, mix together vegetables, beans, and cilantro.
2. In a small bowl, add the ingredients for the dressing.
3. Whisk together the dressing ingredients until blended.
4. Pour dressing onto salad and mix until the dressing is evenly distributed.

Nutrition Facts

- Calories: 247 (12.4%)
- Total Fat: 14.4 g (18%)
- Saturated Fat: 2 g (10%)
- Total Carbohydrates: 26.7 g (10%)
- Dietary Fiber: 7.6 g (27%)
- Protein: 6 g

QUICK TIP

This is a great meal to make ahead because it tastes delicious cold. If you choose to make this meal ahead, we suggest keeping the dressing separate until just before you eat it, as it can make the cilantro soggy. It will store beautifully for up to five days in the fridge.

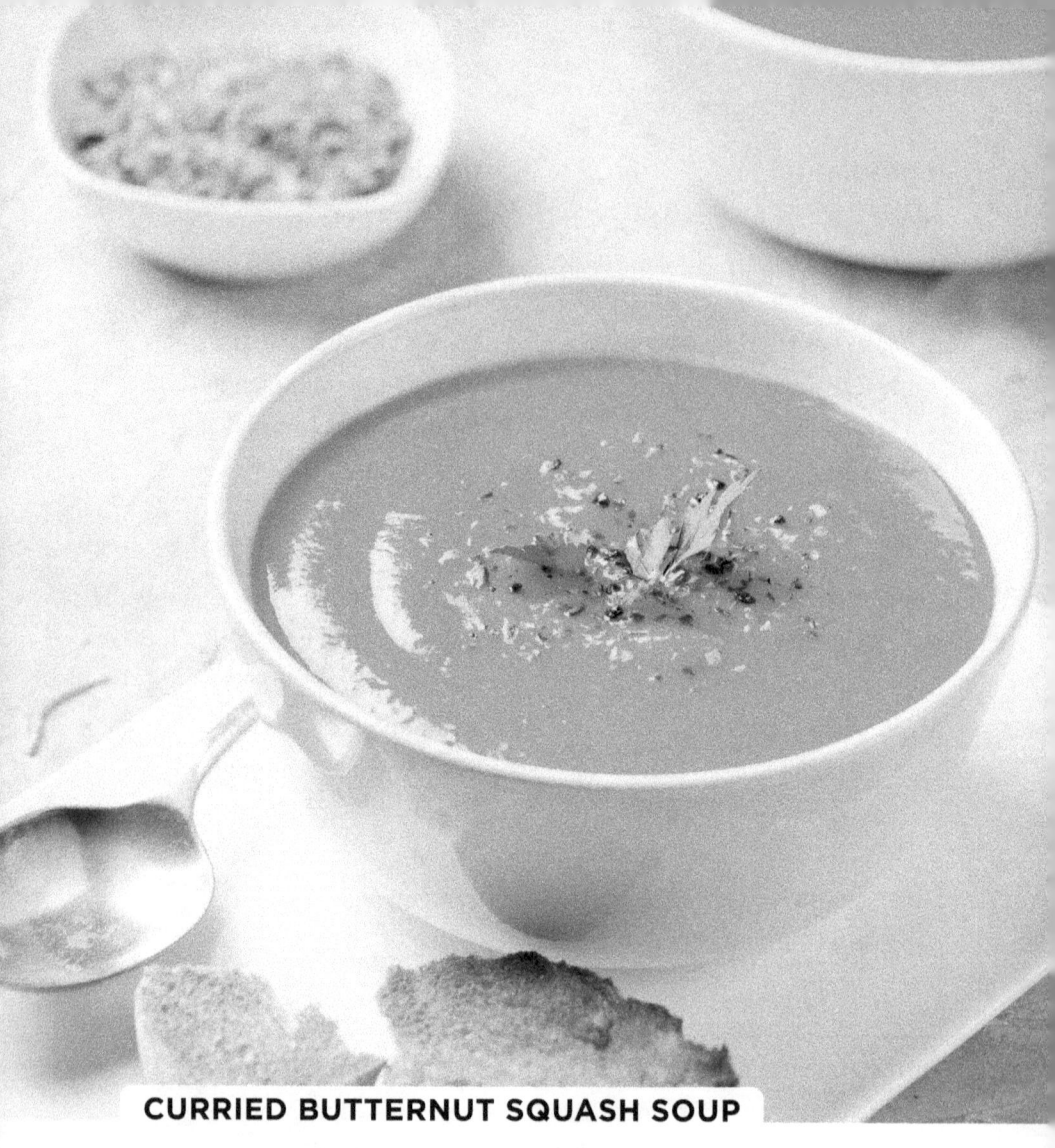

CURRIED BUTTERNUT SQUASH SOUP

Prep time: 15 minutes   Cook time: 25 minutes   Servings: 4

SQUASH IS FOUND IN HUNDREDS of varieties all over the world and is even a staple food in some cultures. Squash is part of the gourd family, and these vegetables contain several components, including beta-carotene, which is linked to a lower risk of developing several types cancers. Nonstarchy vegetables, like squash, are also linked to lower risks of certain types of breast cancer. This recipe uses curry, which not only adds a mouth-watering aroma to the soup but also provides curcumin, a powerful, anti-inflammatory spice.

Ingredients

- 2 tbsp extra virgin olive oil
- 1 cup onion, finely chopped
- 3 cloves garlic, minced
- 4 cups vegetable broth
- 1 butternut squash (or another creamy squash variety you can find locally), cubed, about 5 cups
- 2 tsp curry powder
- ½ tsp ground cumin
- 1 cup nonfat Greek yogurt
- 2 tbsp honey

Nutrition Facts

- Calories: 423 (21.2%)
- Total Fat: 8.8 g (11%)
- Saturated Fat: 1.4 g (7%)
- Total Carbohydrates: 47.6 g (17%)
- Dietary Fiber: 4.6 g (16%)
- Protein: 41.7 g

Directions

1. Add olive oil to a large pot over medium heat. Add onion and garlic and cook until the onion is translucent.
2. Stir in all ingredients except yogurt and honey into the onion mixture. Bring to a boil and simmer for about 10 minutes or until squash is soft.
3. Turn off the heat and use an immersion blender to blend the squash mixture until smooth.
4. Stir in Greek yogurt and honey.
5. Serve hot.

QUICK TIP

This soup recipe freezes beautifully. If you want to make a big batch and save some for later, cool the soup and place it in a freezer-safe tub. It will keep for up to three months!

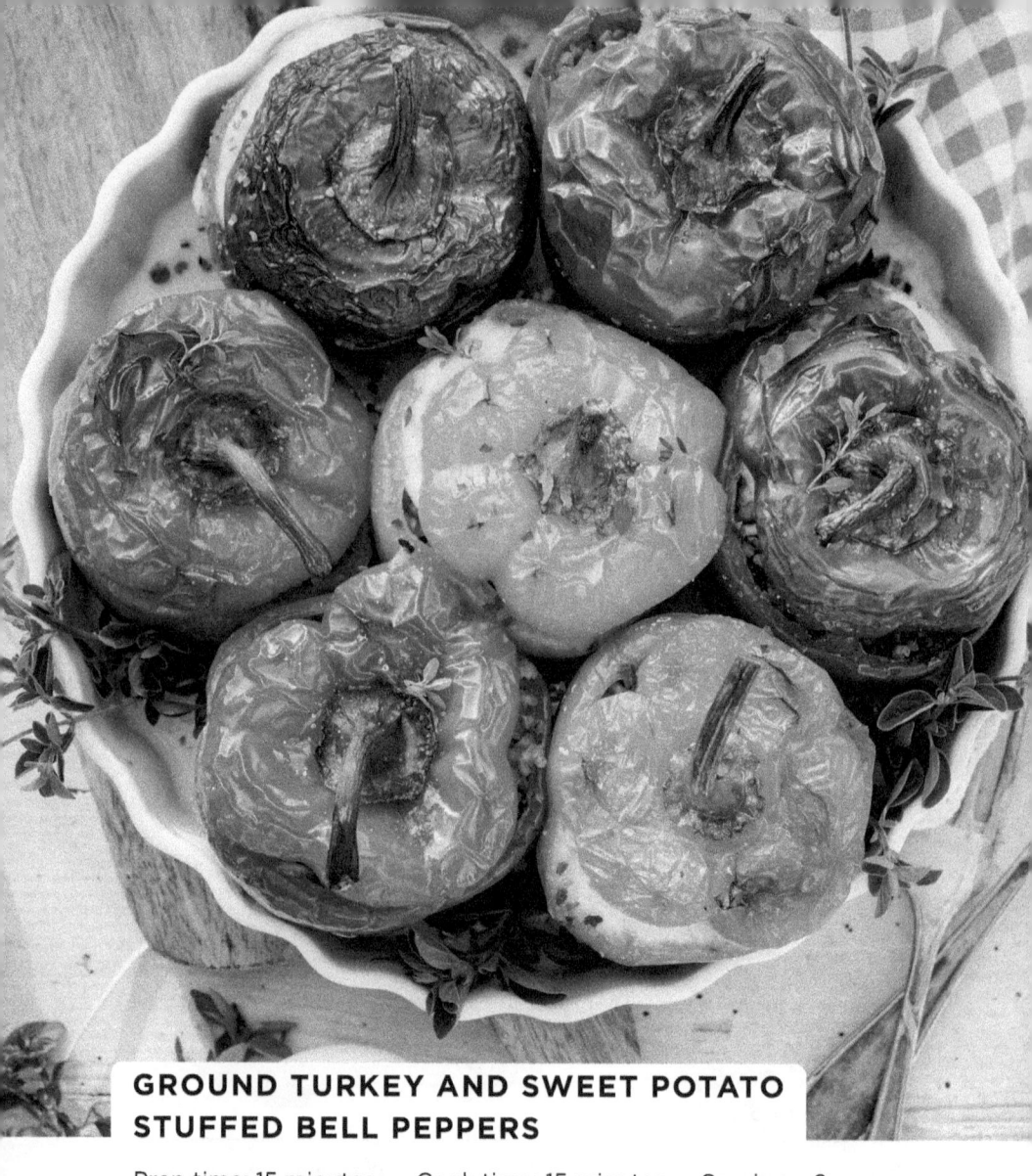

GROUND TURKEY AND SWEET POTATO STUFFED BELL PEPPERS

Prep time: 15 minutes   Cook time: 15 minutes   Servings: 2

THIS MEAL IS PERFECT to enjoy fresh or to make ahead and enjoy the next day. The turkey and sweet potato filling is nourishing and packed with protein and antioxidants. It will also keep you satisfied until your next meal. The bell peppers deliver your recommended daily value of vitamin C, and the sweet potatoes contain antioxidant beta-carotene. The lean ground turkey provides plenty of protein with less saturated fat, which is important for breast health.

Ingredients

- 1 tbsp extra virgin olive oil
- 6 oz lean ground turkey
- 2 cloves garlic
- 1 yellow onion, thinly sliced
- 1 ½ cup sweet potatoes, diced
- ½ cup low sodium tomato sauce
- 2 large bell peppers
- 2 tbsp mozzarella cheese
- 1 tbsp fresh parsley
- Salt and pepper to taste

Directions

1. Preheat oven to 350°F (175°C).
2. Heat the olive oil in a large skillet over medium heat. Use a skillet that has a top.
3. Add the ground turkey, garlic, and onion. Cook until the turkey is browned.
4. Add the sweet potatoes and cover the skillet, stirring every 2–3 minutes. Add about ¼ cup water if the mixture is dry. Cook until the sweet potatoes are tender.
5. Add the tomato sauce, salt, and pepper, and simmer for about 5 minutes.
6. Meanwhile, cut the tops off of the bell peppers and remove the seeds. Place them on a baking dish.
7. Turn off the stovetop and spoon the mixture into each bell pepper until full. Top with mozzarella.
8. Bake uncovered for about 30 minutes.
9. Garnish with parsley and serve hot.

Nutrition Facts

- Calories: 470 (23.5%)
- Total Fat: 18.8 g (24%)
- Saturated Fat: 5.2 g (26%)
- Total Carbohydrates: 48.4 g (18%)
- Dietary Fiber: 5.1 g (18%)
- Protein: 33 g

QUICK TIP

Don't like bell peppers? This filling tastes great inside a whole-wheat wrap, too! Place a large whole-wheat tortilla on a pan in the oven to get it slightly warm before filling your wrap for a delicious and nourishing lunch.

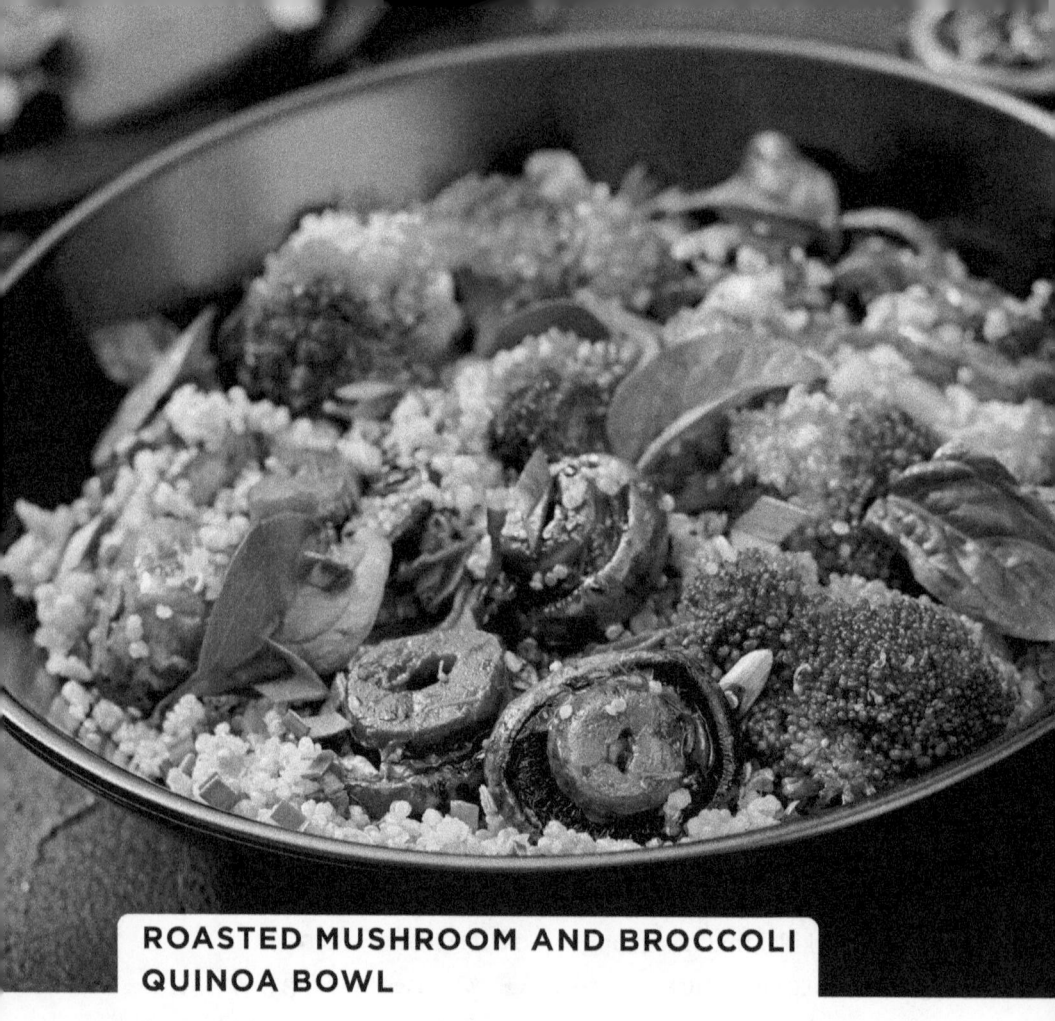

ROASTED MUSHROOM AND BROCCOLI QUINOA BOWL

Prep time: 5 minutes   Cook time: 30 minutes   Servings: 3

QUINOA IS AN INCREDIBLE food. It is a complete protein and a whole grain in one, and it is packed with vitamins and minerals to nourish your body. Here, we've taken the standard quinoa up a notch to boost breast health; we've added broccoli, which contains antioxidant components shown to reduce the risk of breast cancer when consumed regularly, and mushrooms, which contain enzymes that may help regulate the hormones associated with breast cancer. Benefits aside, this is a delicious, filling one-plate meal that can be enjoyed hot or cold.

Ingredients

- 1 cup quinoa
- 2 cups low sodium vegetable broth (or low sodium chicken broth for a nonvegetarian version)
- 1 cup cremini mushrooms, whole
- 2 cups broccoli florets
- 1 tsp dried Italian herbs
- 1 garlic clove, minced
- 3 tbsp olive oil
- Salt and pepper to taste
- Fresh basil for garnishing (optional)

Directions

1. Preheat oven to 400°F (205°C)
2. Pour olive oil on a cookie sheet and then place broccoli florets and mushrooms over the oil.
3. Sprinkle garlic, Italian herbs, and salt and pepper over the broccoli and mushrooms. Shake the cookie sheet to coat the vegetables in oil and spices. Roast in the oven for about 30 minutes.
4. Place vegetable broth in a saucepan over medium heat. When it comes to a boil, pour in quinoa, cover, and let simmer on low for about 15–20 minutes or until fluffy and the white "tail" appears around the quinoa grains.
5. To serve, divide the quinoa among 3 bowls. For presentation, you can spoon the quinoa into half of each bowl and then add the vegetables to fill the other half of the bowls. Garnish with basil, if desired.

Nutrition Facts

- Calories: 367 (18.4%)
- Total Fat: 17.7 g (23%)
- Saturated Fat: 2.4 g (12%)
- Total Carbohydrates: 44.4 g (16%)
- Dietary Fiber: 5.7 g (20%)
- Protein: 10.4 g

QUICK TIP

Are you looking for a nonvegan version of this recipe? You can add some shredded rotisserie chicken or leftover ground turkey to the dish for an easy and quick way to change it up.

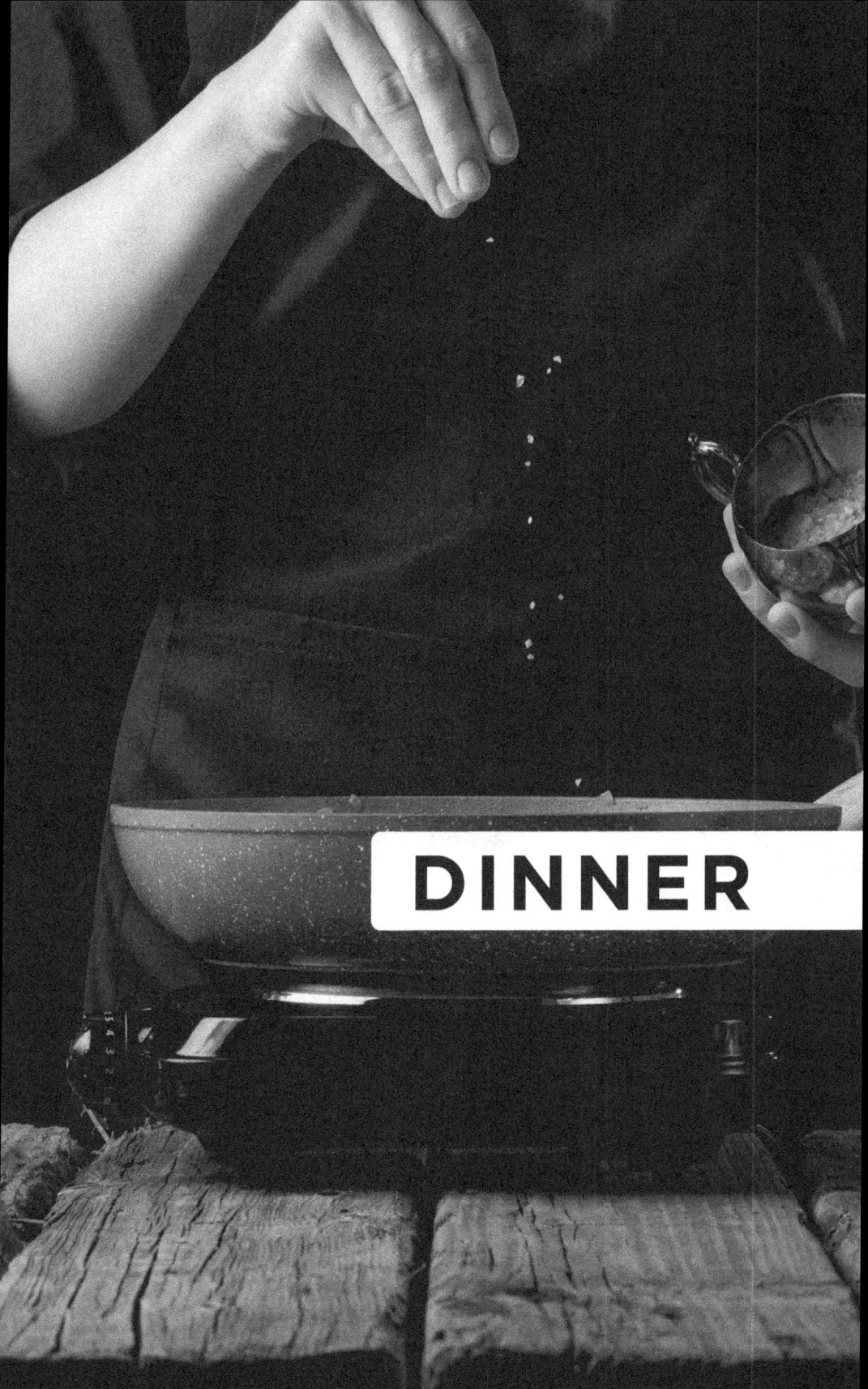

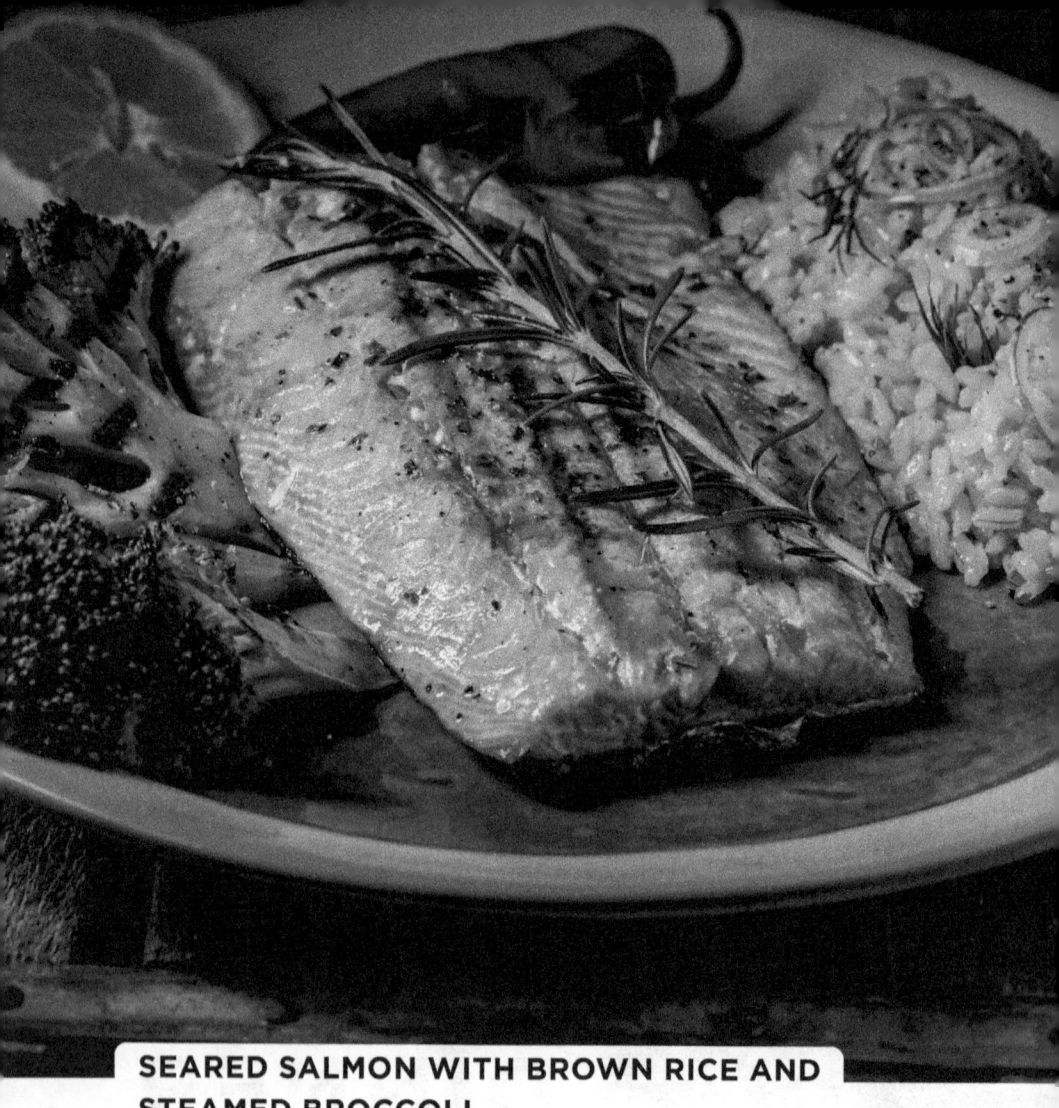

SEARED SALMON WITH BROWN RICE AND STEAMED BROCCOLI

Prep time: 10 minutes   Cook time: 40 minutes   Servings: 4

EACH ELEMENT OF THIS COMPLETE MEAL is packed with nutrients that support breast health. Salmon is one of the types of fish highest in omega-3 fatty acids, which, in addition to being anti-inflammatory, research shows may inhibit the growth of breast tumors when consumed regularly. The brown rice and broccoli contribute whole fiber to the diet, which promotes hormone balance. Not to mention, this delicious and wholesome meal is packed with flavor and will keep you satisfied until your morning meal.

DINNER

Ingredients

- 4 6 oz salmon fillets
- 1 tsp dried thyme
- 2 tsp white wine
- 1 garlic clove, minced
- ½ lemon
- 1 tbsp olive oil
- 1 cup brown rice, rinsed
- 4 cups broccoli florets
- Salt and pepper to taste

Directions

1. Place 2 ½ cups of slightly salted water in a saucepan and bring to a boil.
2. Once boiling, add brown rice. Cover and cook for about 45 minutes or until the rice has absorbed the water.
3. Meanwhile, place raw salmon on a plate and season with salt, pepper, and thyme.
4. Heat olive oil in a skillet and, once hot, add salmon. Add white wine and minced garlic.
5. Cook for about 5 minutes on each side or until flaky. Increase the heat and cook for an additional 1 minute on each side. Set aside.
6. In a vegetable steamer or a saucepan with about ¼ cup boiling water, add broccoli. Cover and steam for about 4 minutes.
7. Plate the salmon, broccoli, and brown rice, and squeeze fresh lemon over the salmon and broccoli.

Nutrition Facts

- Calories: 511 (25.6%)
- Total Fat: 17.1 g (22%)
- Saturated Fat: 3.8 g (19%)
- Total Carbohydrate: 43.4 g (16%)
- Dietary Fiber: 4.3 g (15%)
- Protein: 47.3 g

QUICK TIP

To keep the salmon from sticking to the pan, use a seasoned cast iron pan or a nonstick frying pan in addition to heated oil.

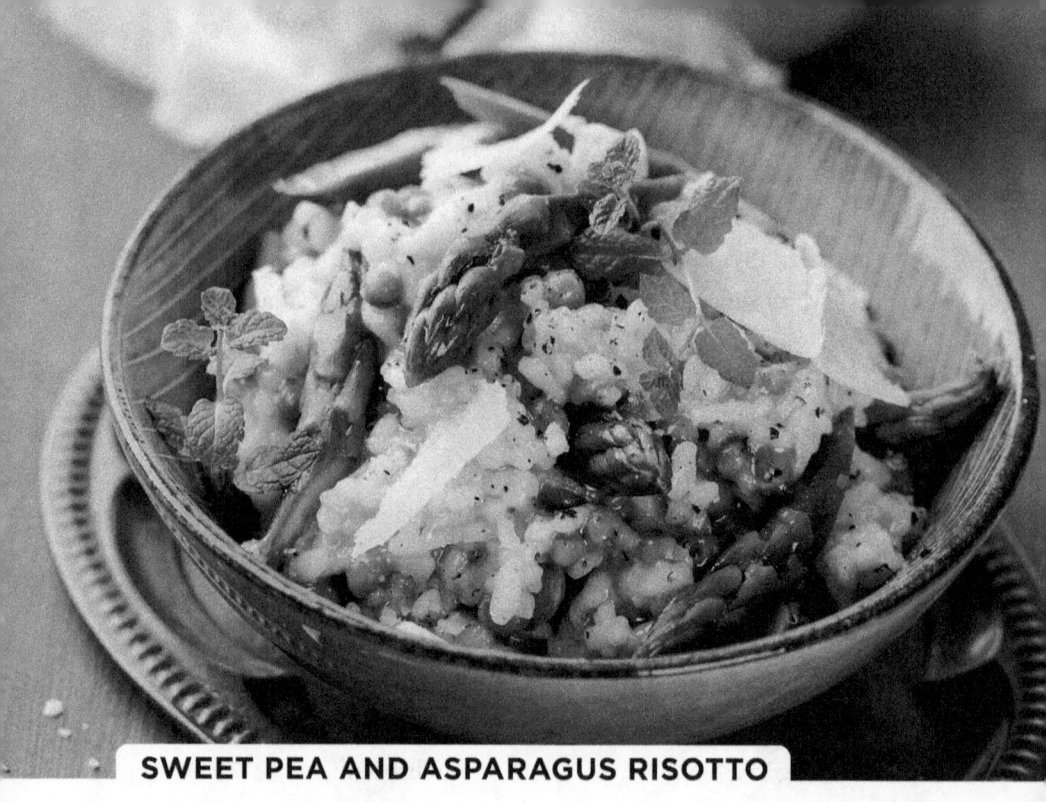

SWEET PEA AND ASPARAGUS RISOTTO

Prep time: 10 minutes   Cook time: 20 minutes   Servings: 4

RISOTTO IS A CLASSIC hearty Italian dish with unlimited possibilities. Here, we've decided to bring peas and asparagus to center stage, both of which are packed with antioxidant compounds like catechin, vitamin C, vitamin E, and various flavonoids and polyphenols to support your immune system. Research shows that women who eat a variety of vegetables have a lower risk of breast cancer and tend to have better outcomes if they do develop breast cancer. Enjoy this sweet pea and asparagus risotto to the very last bite.

Ingredients

- 2 cups frozen peas or fresh cooked peas
- 1 cup fresh asparagus, chopped into 1 cm pieces
- 1 bay leaf
- 2 oz grated parmesan cheese
- ¼ cup olive oil
- 1 shallot, sliced
- 1 cup Arborio rice
- ½ cup dry white wine
- 1 lemon
- ¼ cup fresh parsley, chopped
- Salt and pepper to taste

Directions

1. In large pot, add 5 cups of slightly salted water and bring to a boil. Add peas, asparagus, and bay leaf, and boil for 15 minutes to make stock.
2. Reserve stock and remove peas and asparagus from the pot. Set aside ½ cup peas and asparagus to add to the rice later on.
3. Place the remaining peas and asparagus together with 1 cup stock in a blender and blend to make a puree.
4. In a large pan, heat olive oil on low. Add shallots and a pinch of salt and cook until tender.
5. Add Arborio rice to the pan and stir until browned.
6. Pour in wine with rice until the wine is almost completely evaporated.
7. Add stock to the pan with the rice ½ cup at a time. Stir often and add more when the water is nearly absorbed. Continue until the rice is tender and slightly sticky, which will be after 1 ½ to 2 cups of rice.
8. Add pea puree to the mixture. Cover and simmer for about 5 minutes.
9. Stir in remaining peas, asparagus, and parmesan cheese, and squeeze in the juice from ½ lemon.
10. Divide among 4 bowls and top with fresh parsley, if desired.

Nutrition Facts

- Calories: 394 (19.7%)
- Total Fat: 16.1 g (21%)
- Saturated Fat: 3.9 g (19%)
- Total Carbohydrate: 48.1 g (17%)
- Dietary Fiber: 4.7 g (17%)
- Protein: 10.9 g

QUICK TIP

Avoid overcooking the risotto by slowly adding the stock and waiting until the rice absorbs it. The rice should be soft and tender, but you should still be able to distinguish each rice kernel.

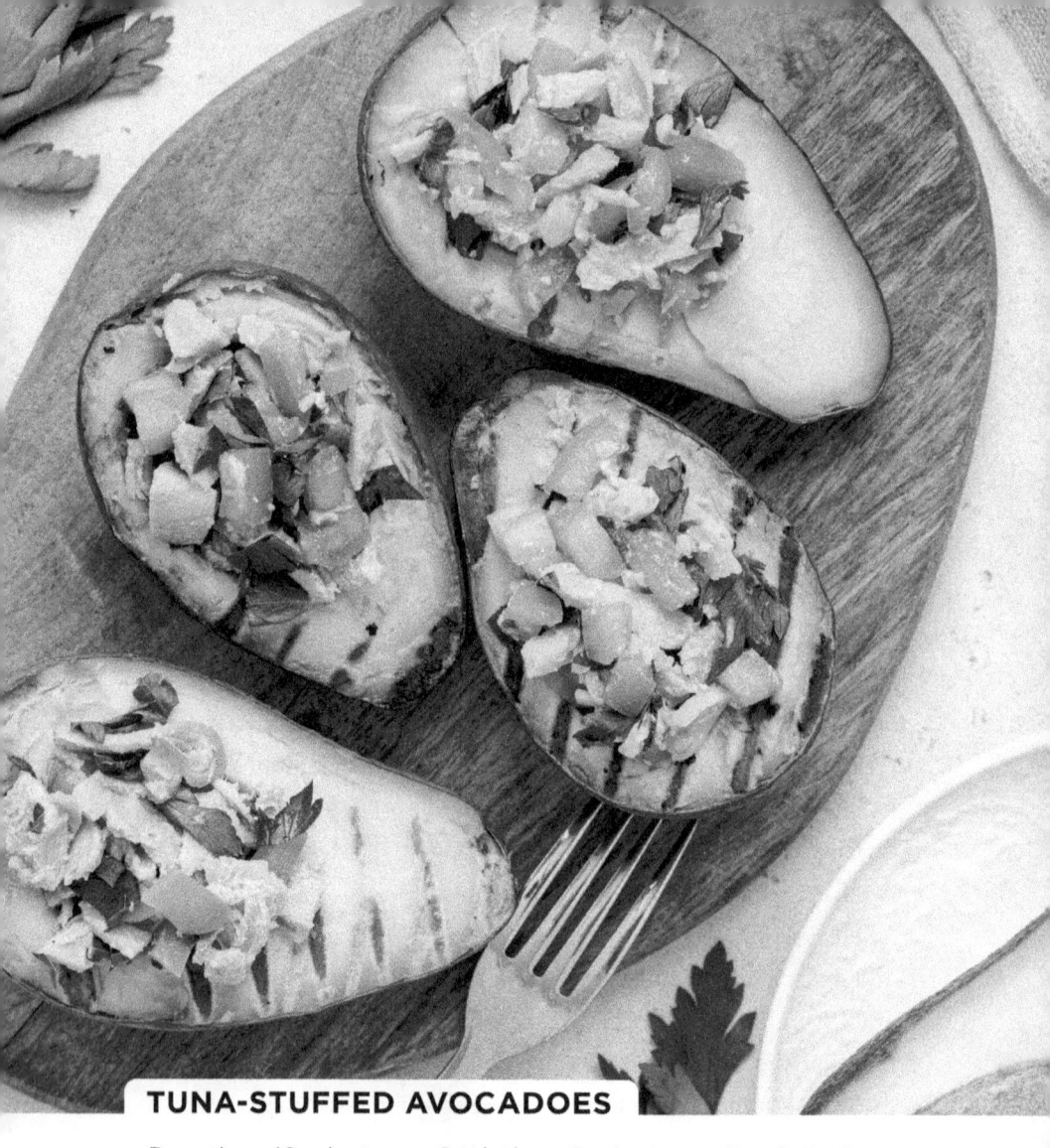

TUNA-STUFFED AVOCADOES

Prep time: 10 minutes   Cook time: 0 minutes   Servings: 2

THIS QUICK AND EASY dinner is packed with anti-inflammatory omega-3 fatty acids and a variety of antioxidants to end your day with the right balance of nutrition. You don't need to cook this meal, and it is ready to be enjoyed in as little as 10 minutes. Enjoy the stuffed avocadoes on their own, or pair with a vegetable soup to add an extra serving or two of vegetables to your day.

Ingredients

- 1 ripe avocado, halved
- 1 can tuna in water, drained
- 2 green onions, chopped
- 1 red bell pepper, chopped
- ¼ cup parsley, chopped
- Juice from ½ lime
- 2 tbsp light mayonnaise
- Salt and pepper to taste

Directions

1. In a small bowl, mix the tuna, green onions, bell pepper, parsley, lime, and mayonnaise. Add salt and pepper to taste.
2. Cut the avocado in half and remove the pit.
3. Spoon tuna salad into the avocado and serve.

Nutrition Facts

- Calories: 402 (20.1%)
- Total Fat: 27.3 g (35%)
- Saturated Fat: 5.5 g (28%)
- Total Carbohydrate: 19.1 g (7%)
- Dietary Fiber: 8.2 g (29%)
- Protein: 23.5 g

QUICK TIP

For a heartier, warm version of this recipe, heat up the oven to 350°F (170°C), and place a thin slice of swiss cheese on top of the avocado. Place in the oven for 8–10 minutes or until the cheese is melted and slightly brown, and enjoy!

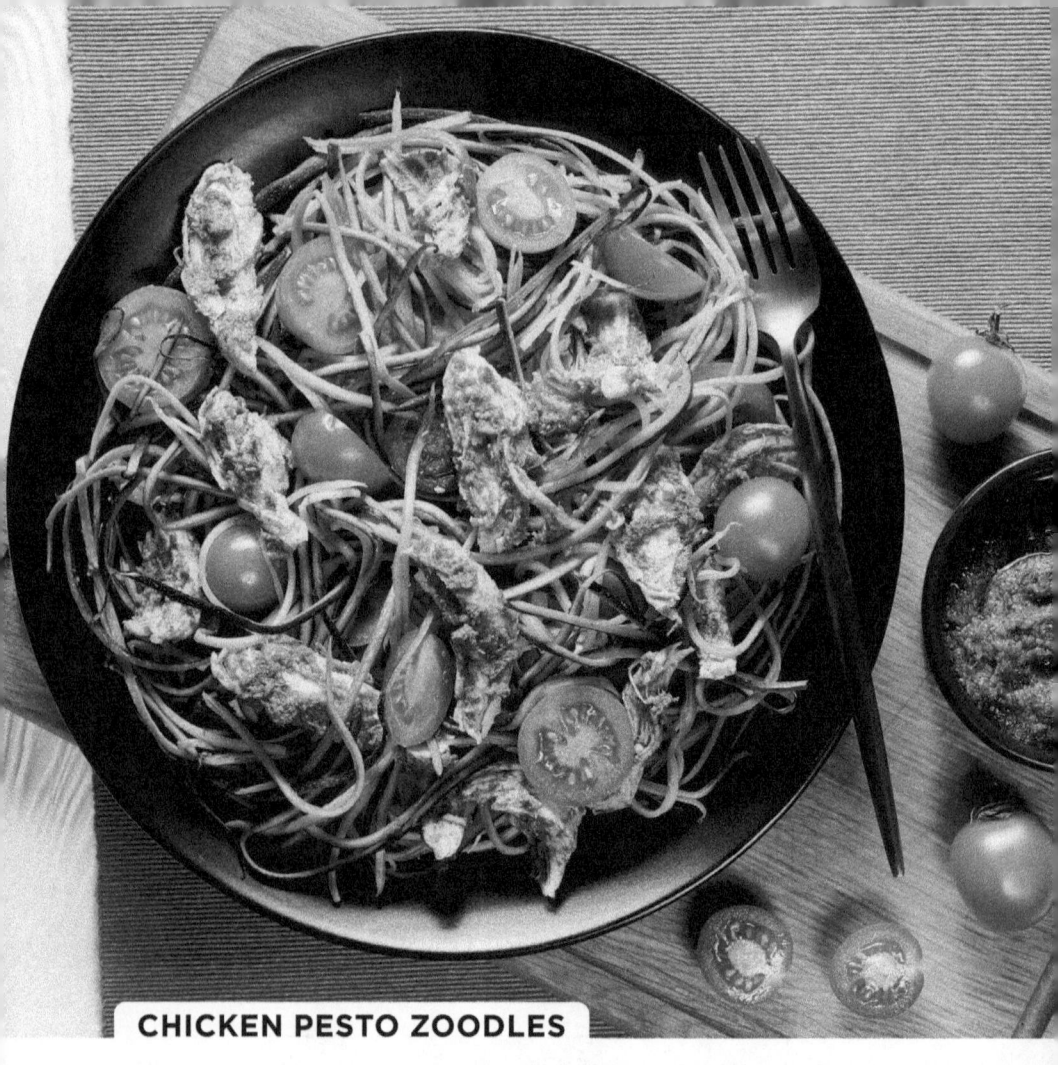

CHICKEN PESTO ZOODLES

Prep time: 15 minutes   Cook time: 15 minutes   Servings: 3

THERE IS NOTHING WRONG with traditional pasta, but zucchini noodles help us get some added veggies into our meals with the breast-health-promoting nutrients that come along with them. The zucchinis in this recipe contain antioxidant phenolic compounds, and basil is a powerhouse herb with a variety of health-promoting properties, including antioxidants like lutein and beta-carotene that reduce inflammation and oxidative stress and a variety of phytochemicals that help to prevent several types of cancer. The pine nuts and olive oil provide healthy, anti-inflammatory fats, and the chicken adds lean protein; together, these make the chicken more satisfying.

DINNER

Ingredients

- 1 large zucchini
- 1 cup fresh basil leaves
- ¼ cup olive oil
- 2 tbsp pine nuts
- 3 tbsp grated parmesan cheese
- ½ cup cherry tomatoes, halved
- 6 oz chicken breast
- Salt and pepper to taste

Directions

1. Using a spiralizer, cut up the zucchini into noodles.
2. Using a steamer, cook the zucchini until tender, about 4–5 minutes.
3. Place basil, olive oil, pine nuts, and parmesan cheese into a food processor. Blend until paste-like.
4. Season raw chicken breast with salt and pepper. Heat a drizzle of olive oil in a nonstick pan on medium heat. Place chicken breast onto the pan and cook for about 7–10 minutes on each side or until cooked through and juices run clear.
5. Using forks, shred the chicken.
6. In a large bowl, mix together the zoodles, pesto, fresh tomatoes, and chicken. Serve hot.

Nutrition Facts

- Calories: 492 (24.6%)
- Total Fat: 28.6 g (37%)
- Saturated Fat: 4.1 g (20%)
- Total Carbohydrate: 6.1 g (2%)
- Dietary Fiber: 2.3 g (7%)
- Protein: 53.1 g

QUICK TIP

Don't have a spiralizer? No problem! You can cut the zucchini lengthwise into strips that are about ½ cm wide and thick. No need to peel the zucchini; the peel adds fiber and contains several antioxidant compounds.

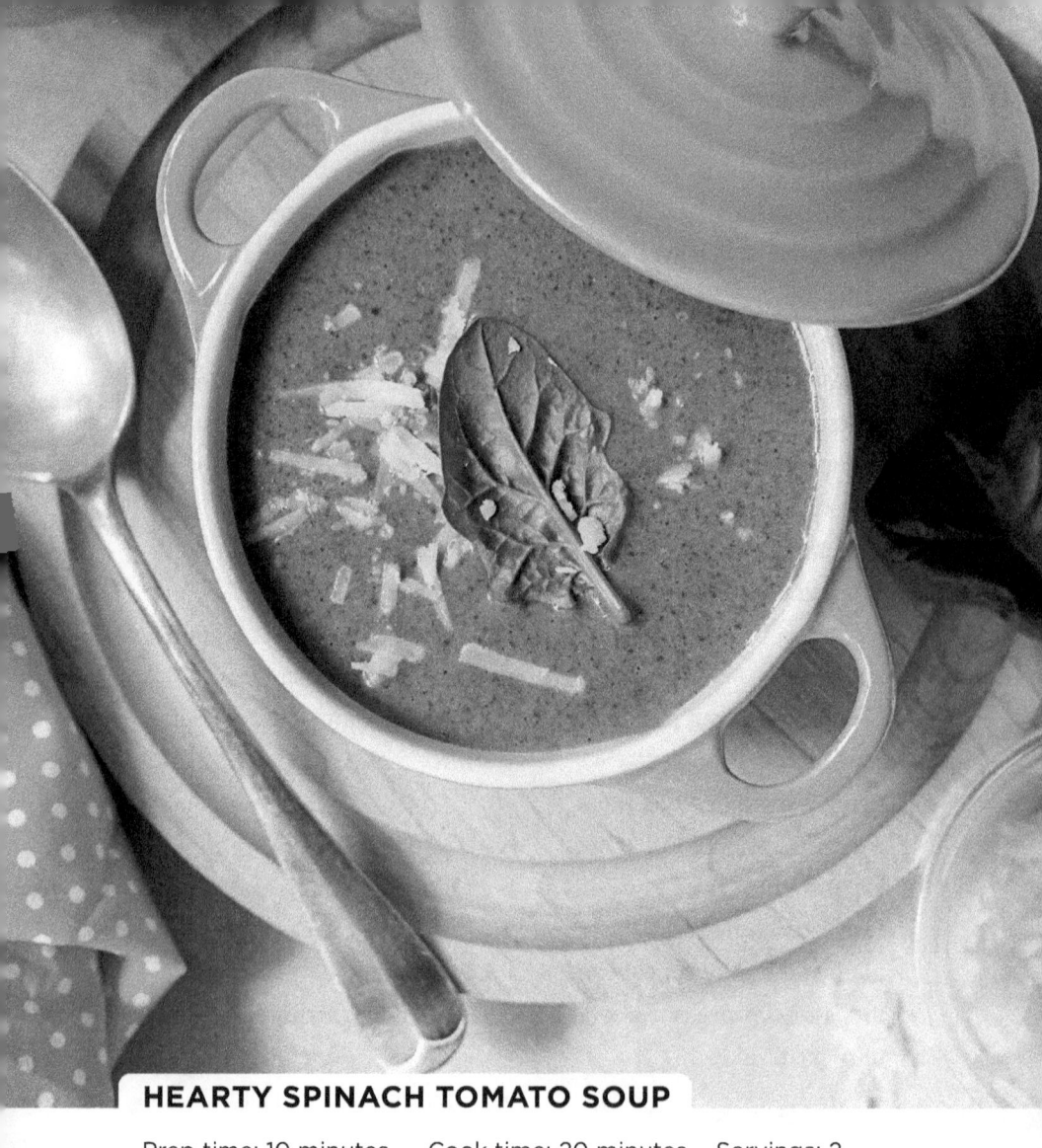

HEARTY SPINACH TOMATO SOUP

Prep time: 10 minutes   Cook time: 20 minutes   Servings: 2

WHEN YOU'RE HUNGRY, THERE'S nothing like a hearty soup to fill your belly. Potatoes are a great source of vitamin C and carotenoids, which are powerful antioxidant compounds. Spinach is often considered a "superfood" because it is rich in vitamins, minerals, and phenolic compounds that support your health, including your breast health. Enjoy this soup on its own, or pair it with the stuffed avocado recipe we shared above.

Ingredients

- 2 cups cubed red potatoes (keep peel on) (about 2 medium potatoes)
- 1 tablespoon dried onion flakes
- 1 ½ cup chicken broth (or vegetable broth for a vegetarian version)
- ½ teaspoon garlic salt
- 2 cups spinach, chopped thinly
- 1 cup low fat Greek yogurt
- ¼ tsp nutmeg

Directions

1. In a large pot, combine chicken broth, potatoes, and onion. Cook for about 10 minutes or until tender.
2. Stir in the remaining ingredients and simmer for about 4–5 minutes or until the spinach is wilted.
3. Using an immersion blender, blend until the soup is smooth.
4. Add yogurt and remove from heat. Divide among 2 bowls and enjoy.

Nutrition Facts

- Calories: 287 (14.6%)
- Total Fat: 3.8 g (5%)
- Saturated Fat: 2.1 g (11%)
- Total Carbohydrate: 42.9 g (16%)
- Dietary Fiber: 4.1 g (15%)
- Protein: 20.3 g

QUICK TIP

If you want to add some more texture to the soup, you can add ¼ cup of quinoa to each serving and stir it in. Quinoa will also add some plant-based protein and fiber to the mix.

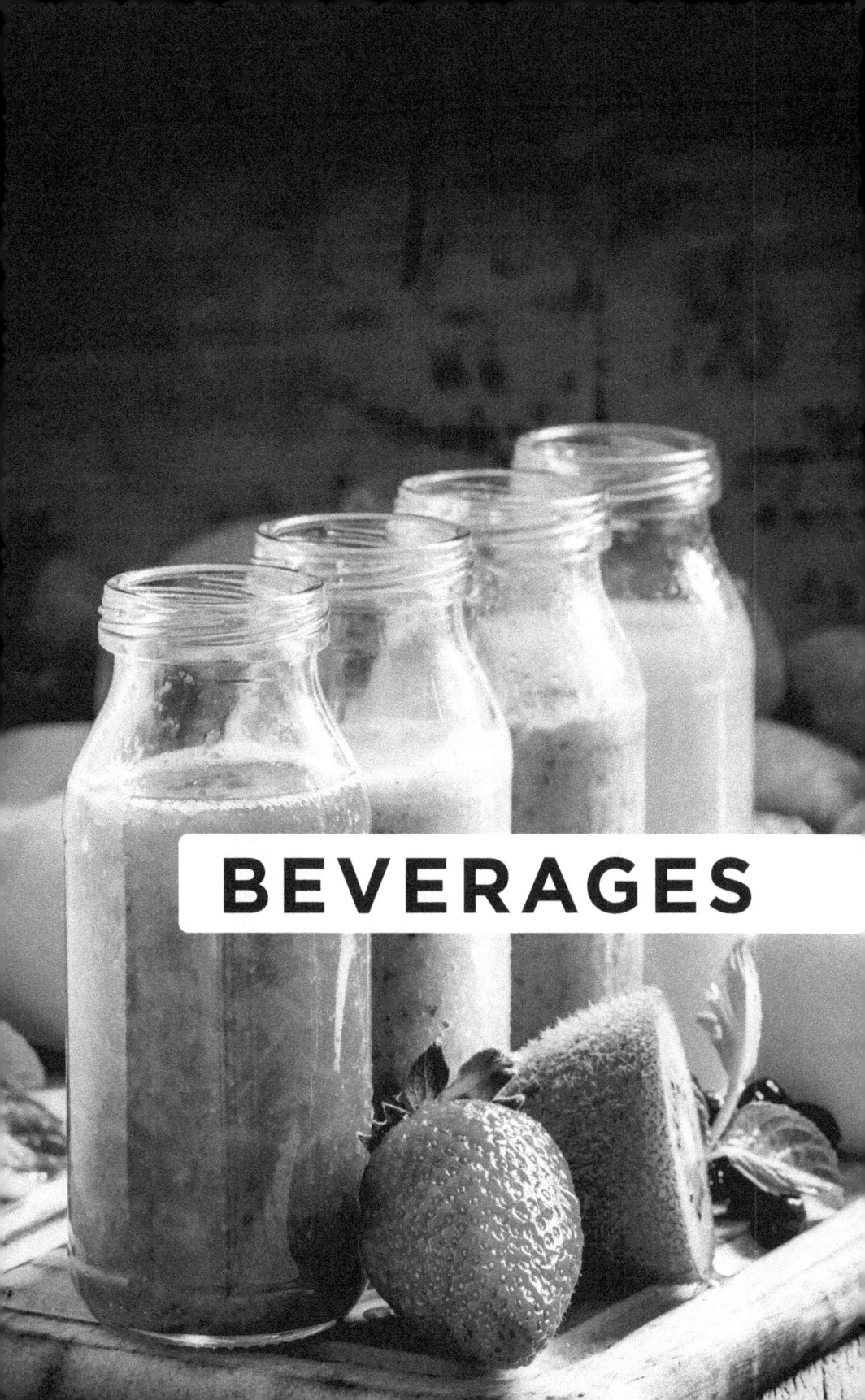

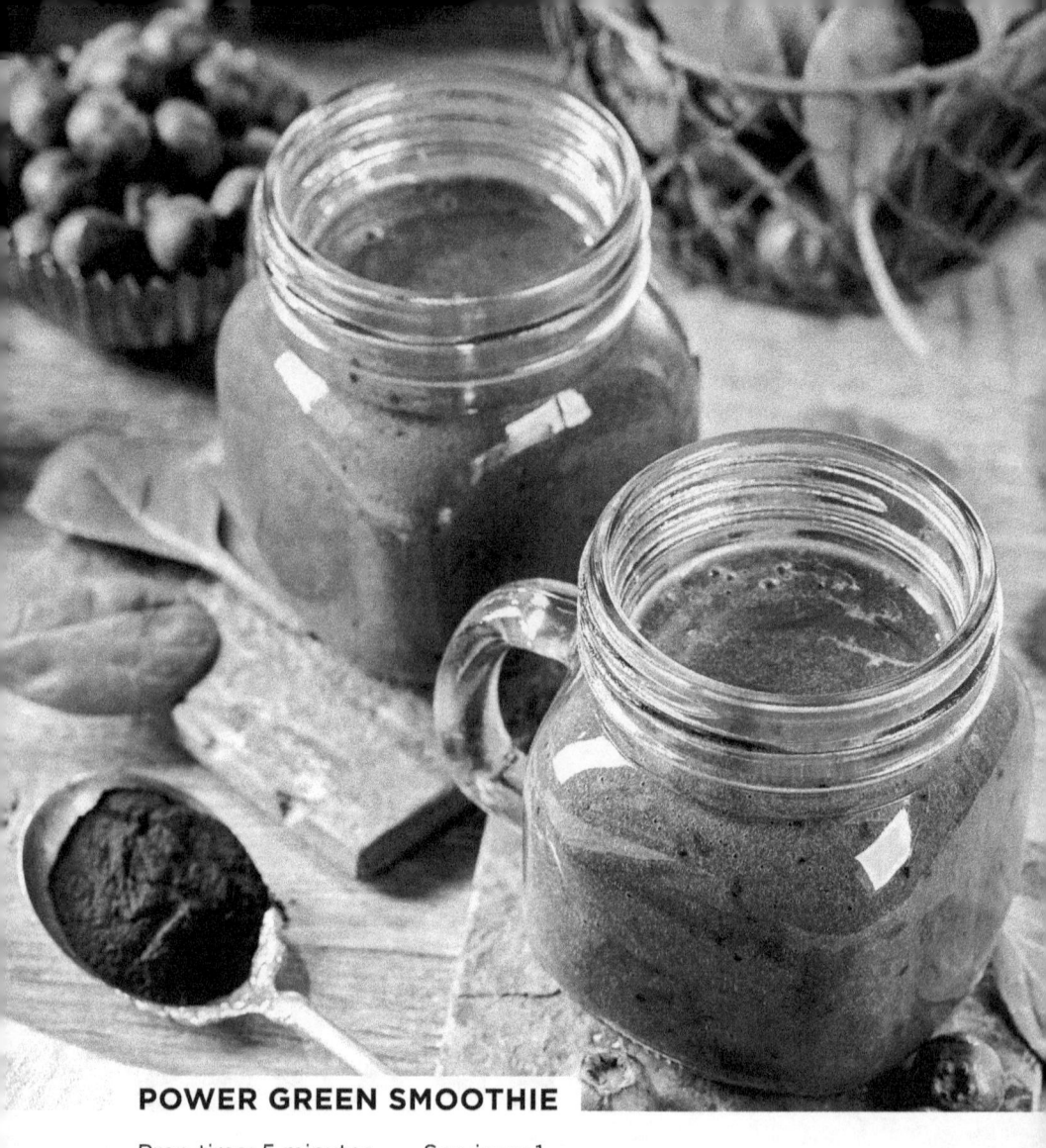

POWER GREEN SMOOTHIE

Prep time: 5 minutes   Servings: 1

THIS SMOOTHIE IS FAST AND EASY to make and is a great way to get some fruits, vegetables, healthy fats, and protein in your diet at any time of day. If you've never tried spinach in a smoothie before, you'll be happy to know the fruits make it so that you barely taste the green leafies. Instead you taste the tropical fruits and the nutty notes of the almonds. The fruits and vegetables provide plenty of antioxidants, while the almonds deliver anti-inflammatory omega-3 fatty acids and plant-based protein.

Ingredients
- 1 cup spinach
- 1 cup skim milk, almond milk, or other plant-based beverage
- ½ cup green grapes
- ½ cup pineapple
- ¼ cup almonds
- ¼ cup blueberries

Directions
Put all ingredients in a blender, and blend until smooth.

Nutrition Facts
One serving of the smoothie made with 1 cup skim milk provides:
- Calories: 323 (16.2%)
- Total Fat: 12.8 g (16%)
- Saturated Fat: 1.3 g (6%)
- Total Carbohydrate: 42 g (15%)
- Dietary Fiber: 6.1 g (22%)
- Protein: 15.2 g

QUICK TIP

Depending on your personal preferences, you can choose what type of milk to add to your smoothie.

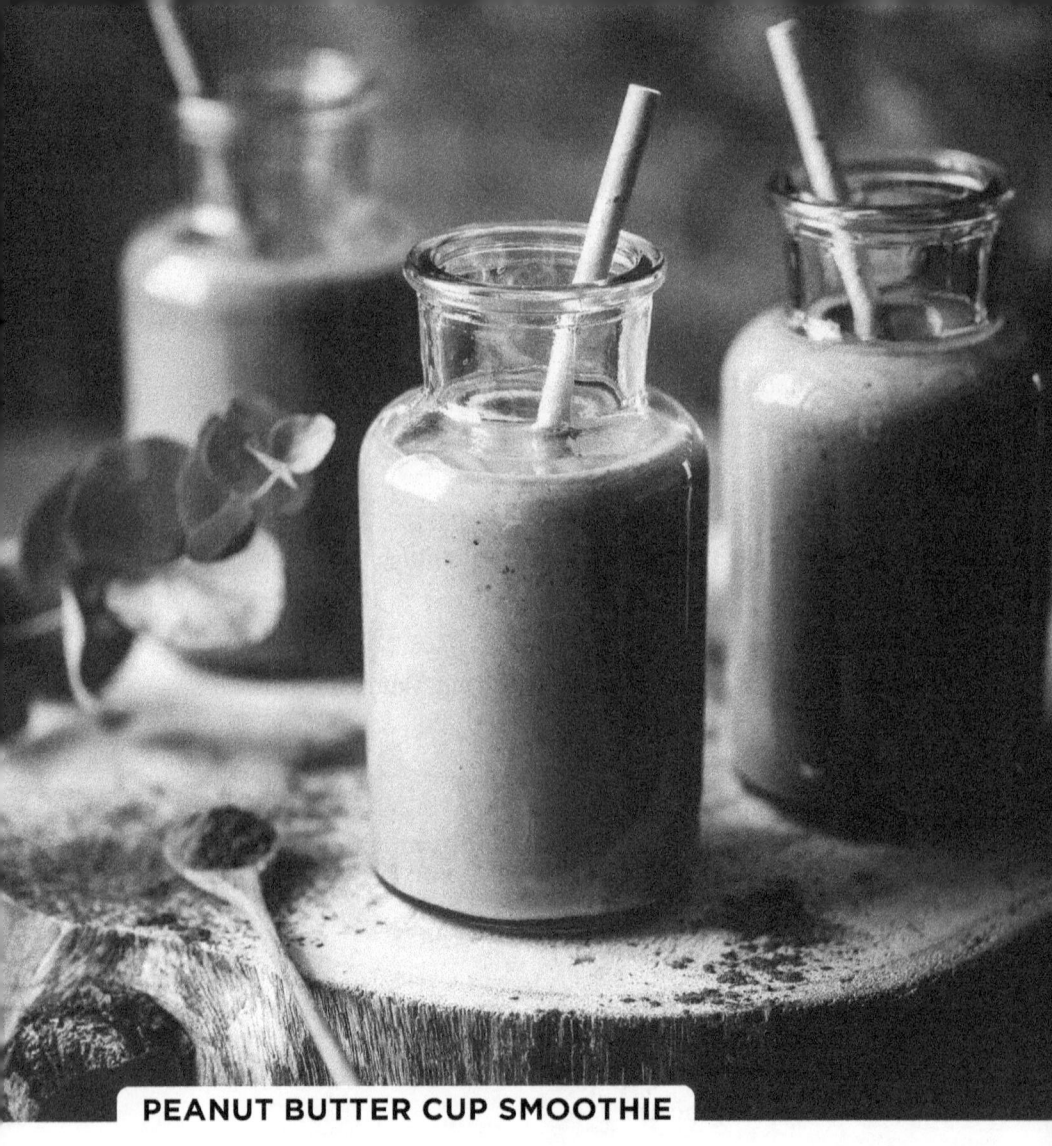

PEANUT BUTTER CUP SMOOTHIE

Prep time: 5 minutes   Servings: 2

DO YOU NEED A PICK-ME-UP for those sweet cravings? Or a dessert you can feel good about? This sweet smoothie is even better than candy because it tastes great and has no added sugar. The nut butter and almonds add protein and anti-inflammatory fats, the yogurt provides protein, the bananas deliver fiber and micronutrients, and the cinnamon provides inflammatory components for women who want a breast-healthy treat.

Ingredients

- ¾ cup low fat Greek yogurt
- 1 cup milk or plant-based milk
- ¼ cup peanut butter
- ¼ cup almonds
- 1 banana (ideally sliced and frozen)
- 1 tsp cinnamon

Directions

Put all ingredients in a blender, and blend until smooth.

Nutrition Facts

One serving of the smoothie made with skim milk provides:

- Calories: 422 (21.1%)
- Total Fat: 24.1 g (26%)
- Saturated Fat: 5.2 g (26%)
- Total Carbohydrate: 32.7 g (12%)
- Dietary Fiber: 5.6 g (20%)
- Protein: 23.9 g

QUICK TIP

Frozen bananas put the "smooth" in smoothie. If you don't have frozen bananas, you can add a handful of ice to give the smoothie a better texture.

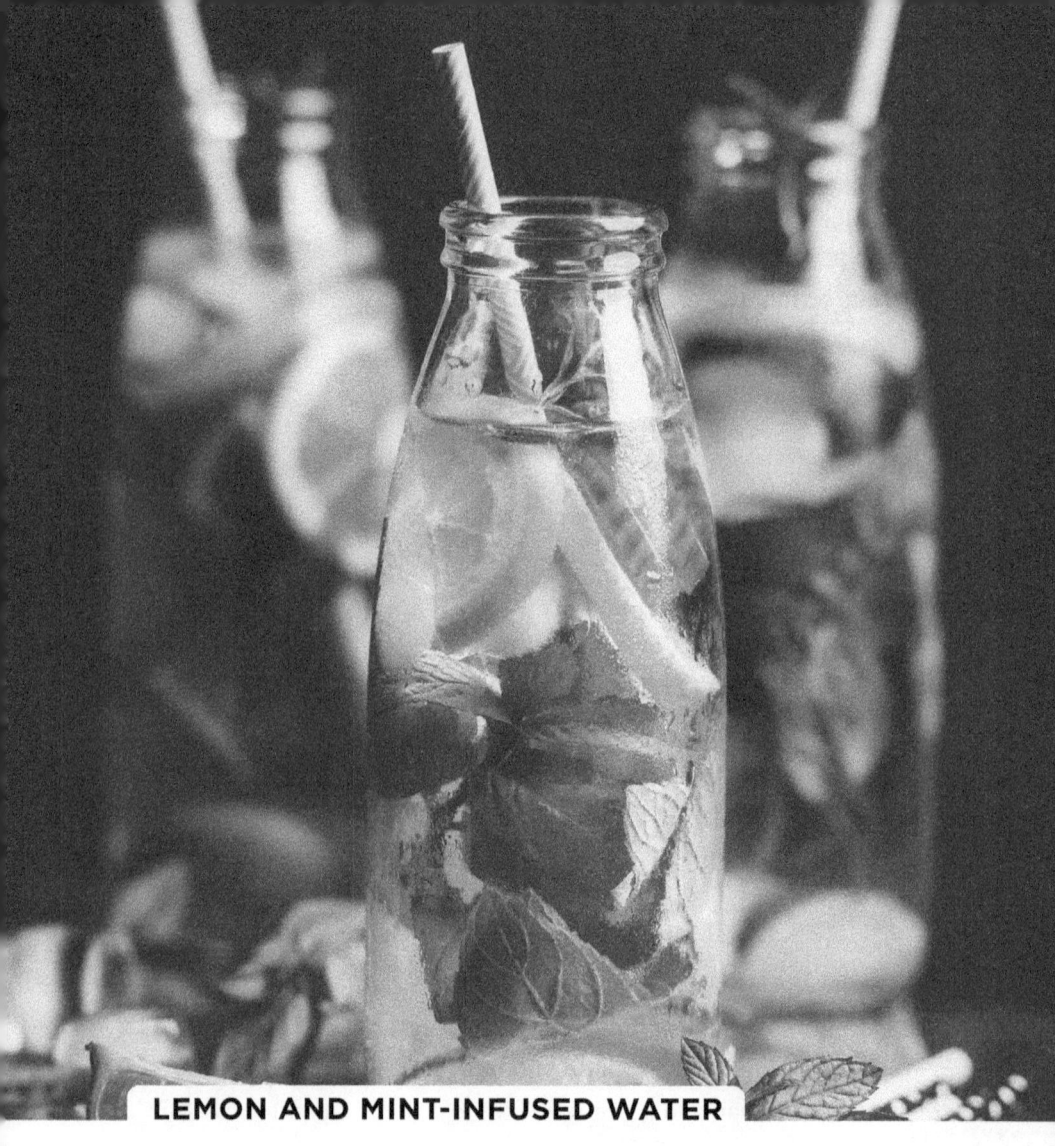

LEMON AND MINT-INFUSED WATER

Prep time: 10 minutes   Cook time: 4 hours   Servings: 4

STAYING HYDRATED IS A VITAL PART of maintaining overall health. However, many of us don't have the habit of drinking water, or we simply don't like the taste of water on its own. This lemon and mint-infused water will make drinking water a whole new experience. It has no added sugar, provides vitamin C and antioxidants, and will help keep you hydrated.

BEVERAGES

Ingredients
- 1 liter water
- 1 lemon, sliced
- ¼ cup mint leaves

Directions
1. In a pitcher of water, add the lemon slices and mint leaves.
2. Place in the refrigerator for at least 4 hours to let the ingredients infuse. Ideally, you can let the water sit overnight.

Nutrition Facts
- Calories: 7 (less than 1%)
- Total Fat: 0.1 g (0%)
- Saturated Fat: 0 g (0%)
- Total Carbohydrate: 1.8 g (1%)
- Dietary Fiber: 0.8 g (3%)
- Protein: 0.4 g

QUICK TIP

Feel free to munch on the mint leaves and lemon for added vitamins, minerals, and antioxidants!

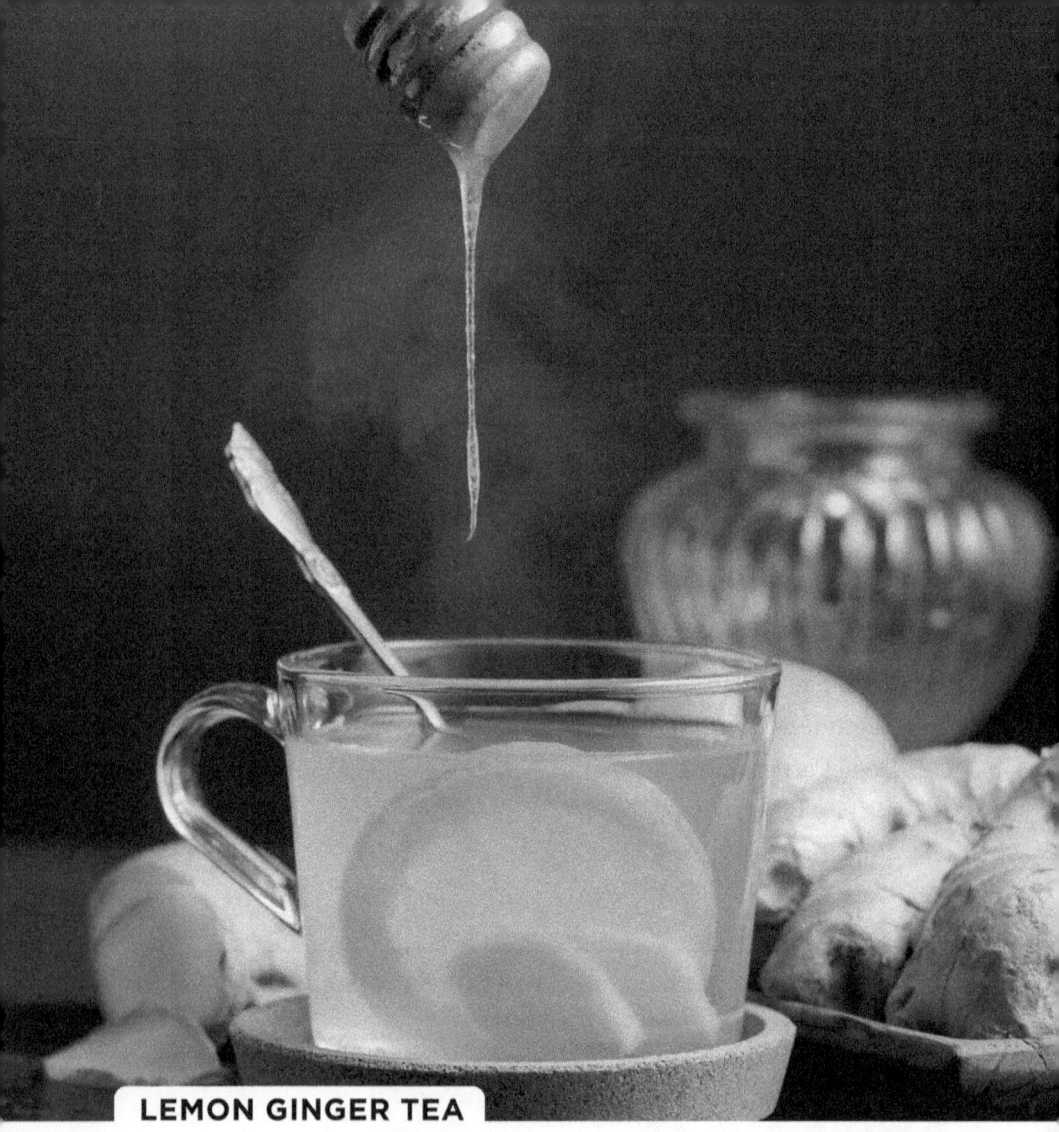

LEMON GINGER TEA

Prep time: 10 minutes   Servings: 4

WE HAD TO ADD A HOT BEVERAGE to our list of recipes because we are fans of cozying up with a warm cup at the end of the day. We love this tea because it is homemade—no need for teabags—and because, while you are sipping on this tasty tea, you'll be putting some powerful anti-inflammatory and antioxidant compounds in your body.

Ingredients
- 1 liter water
- 1 lemon, sliced
- 2 tbsp ginger, grated
- Pure stevia powder to taste (optional)

Directions
1. Place water in a pot and bring to a boil.
2. Once boiling, add lemon and ginger and boil for 1 minute.
3. Turn off and let sit for 5 minutes.
4. Add stevia, if you wish, and enjoy!
5. Enjoy!

Nutrition Facts
- Calories: 13 (less than 1%)
- Total Fat: 0.2 g (0%)
- Saturated Fat: 0.1 g (0%)
- Total Carbohydrate: 3 g (1%)
- Dietary Fiber: 0.4 g (1%)
- Protein: .03 g

QUICK TIP

Ginger and lemon are both digestive aids, so this is a great beverage to drink after a meal.

If you or someone you know is going through chemotherapy, drinking ginger tea may help to manage some of the side effects, like nausea and vomiting.

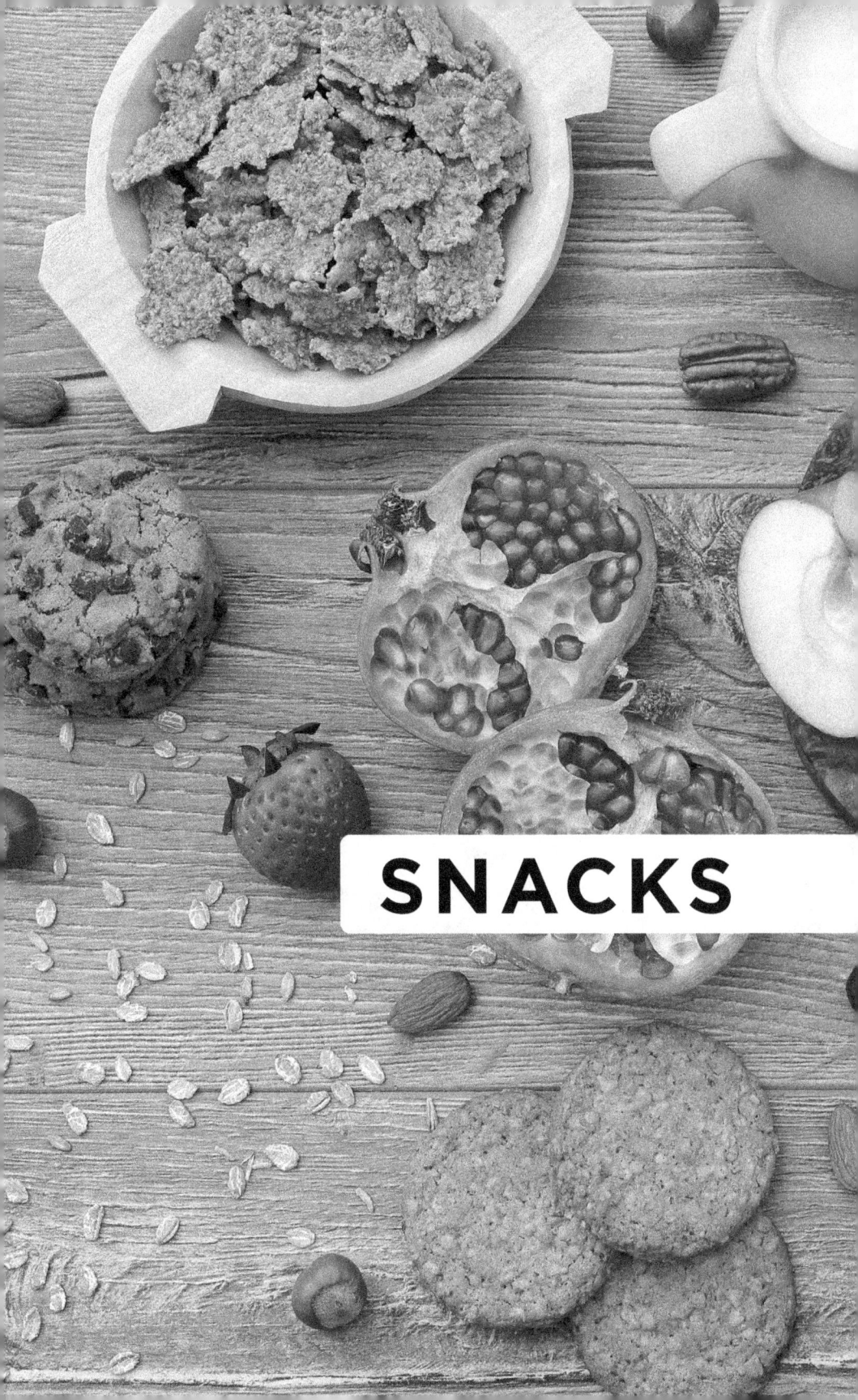
SNACKS

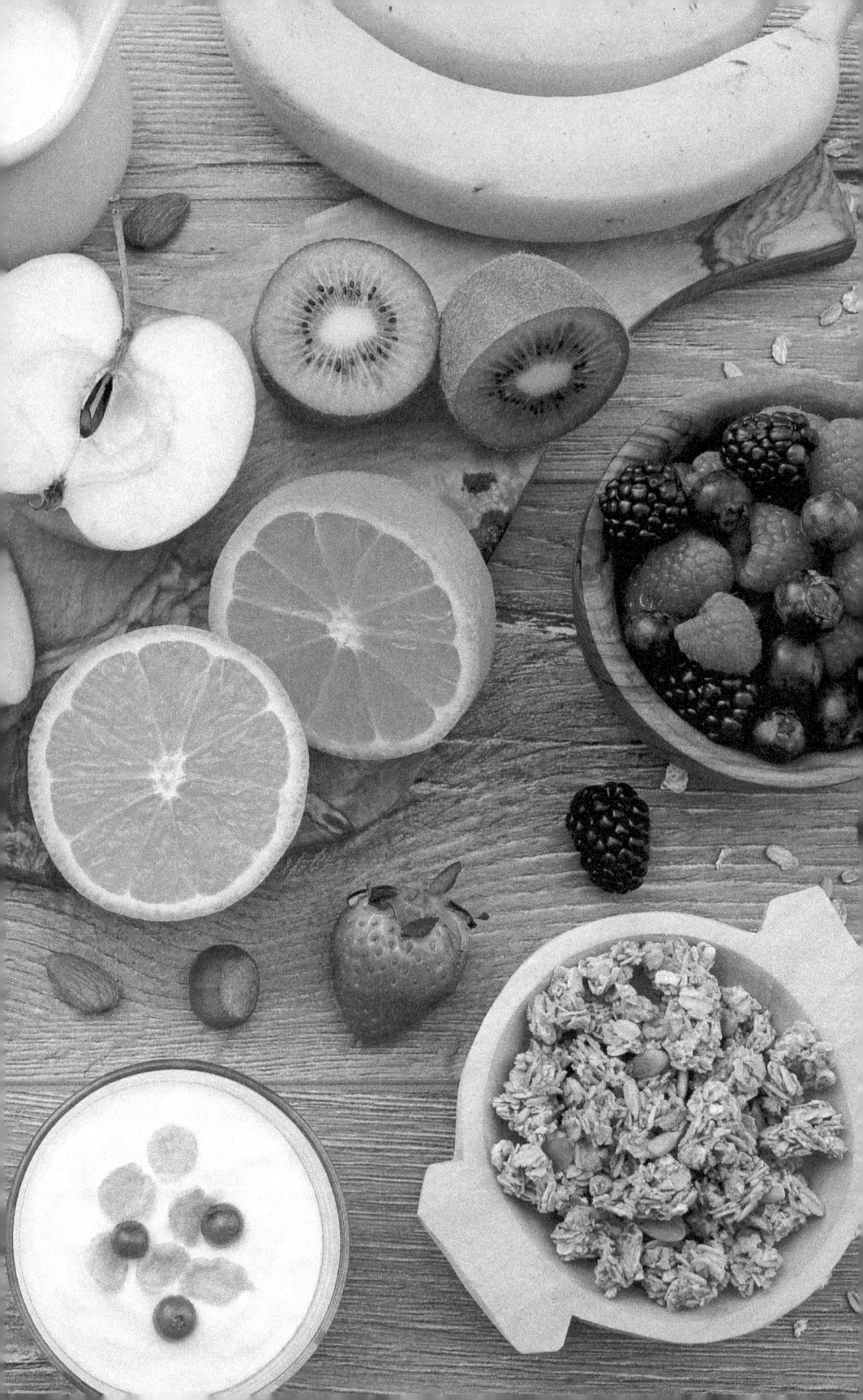

SNACKS ARE AN IMPORTANT PART of many people's lifestyle and daily nutritional needs. They help you refuel between meals, and they also give you an opportunity to get important nutrients into your body.

Most people don't have the time to prepare complicated snacks in the kitchen in addition to cooking meals, so, in this section, we've provided several ideas for grab-and go snacks that include nutrient-dense foods high in antioxidant and anti-inflammatory components that support breast health.

1. **Veggie sticks and hummus:** Raw vegetables contain tons of vitamin C, an antioxidant vitamin that is often lost in the cooking process. Hummus is high in fiber and healthy fats and is a great alternative to creamy dips high in saturated fat.

2. **Natural almond butter and celery:** This is a great snack for when hunger hits in the middle of the day. Take celery sticks, which are high in fiber, to scoop up the almond butter, which is high in anti-inflammatory omega-3 fatty acids, and you're good to go.

3. **Guacamole and chips:** Whip up some guacamole by mixing together avocado, onion flakes, lime, and salt to taste, and you've got yourself an omega-3-packed dip. Pair the guacamole with some low-sodium chips or toasted corn tortillas, and you have a great savory snack.

4. **Banana slices on whole-wheat toast with cinnamon and a drizzle of honey:** For those sweet cravings, you need something sweet! You can whip up this fiber- and mineral-packed snack in as little as 3 minutes. Sprinkle with chia seeds for an extra boost!

5. **Trail mix with dried fruit and nuts:** Nuts are a great source of healthy, anti-inflammatory fats, and dried fruit contains most of the nutrients that fresh fruit does. Aim to find unsweetened dried fruit when possible.

6. **Fruit and yogurt:** Take a cup or bowl of your favorite fruit and pair it with some natural, no-sugar-added yogurt for a complete snack.

7. **Hard-boiled egg and whole-grain crackers:** Hard-boiled eggs are so underrated. Eggs contain complete protein, antioxidant minerals, essential vitamins, and a good balance of fats. They're easy to make ahead and store well in the fridge. Pair a hard-boiled egg with some whole-grain crackers for some added fiber and energy.

8. **Dark chocolate and raspberries:** Need an antioxidant boost? This snack will do it for you. Dark chocolate and raspberries have both been called "superfoods" due to the variety of antioxidants, inflammatory components, vitamins, minerals, and phenolic compounds they contain.

9. **Cottage cheese and pineapple:** Cottage cheese is a great source of calcium, which is important for women's health in general, and just one cup of pineapple delivers more than 100 percent of the recommended daily intake of vitamin C, an important antioxidant vitamin.

10. **Edamame and spices:** Thaw some frozen edamame in the microwave and sprinkle with some spices of your choice. Edamame is high in protein and contains compounds that may help to regulate female hormones.

FINAL THOUGHTS

In this recipe book, we've shared some of our favorite recipes with you. The ingredients were carefully chosen to help support your breast health, but the ingredients will also support most people's overall health. That means that everyone in your family will enjoy them and benefit from them.

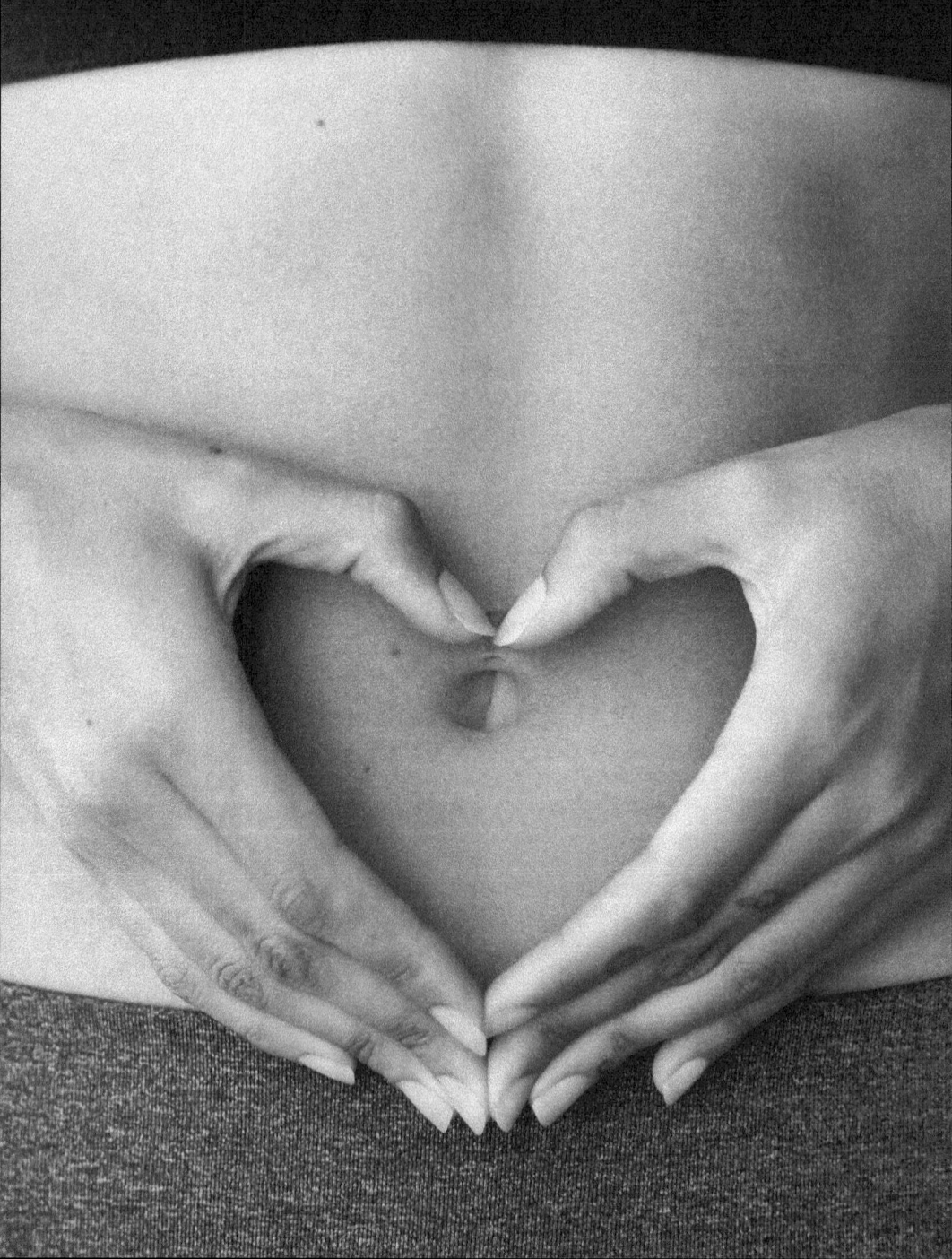

SECTION 5
FITNESS FOR OPTIMAL BREAST HEALTH

EXERCISE

LOVE IT OR HATE IT, the fact (and you know this) is that daily body movement keeps you well and healthy. It fights malignancies, improves treatment outcome, and obviously improves your health and well-being in general.

A significant number of medical and scientific research conducted over the past two decades consistently indicated that an increase in physical activity lowers one's breast cancer risk in many ways.

According to the American Cancer Society, while it is not yet fully known how exercising lowers your risk of breast cancer, it's understood that physical activity boosts your immune function, wards off obesity (being obese raises cancer risk factor), and helps the body regulate hormones including estrogen and insulin (increased levels of these hormones can fuel breast cancer growth).

Research indicates that women who exercise daily are 25 percent less likely to develop breast cancer than those who just sit idly by.

Furthermore, fitness routines are also now infused into cancer patients' care because exercise is believed to help combat not only the physical but also the mental deterioration that usually arises during anti- cancer treatments.

The exercises included in this section are all routines that do not need you to go to the gym or have expensive fitness equipment.

There are definitely many good reasons to spend money for a gym membership and fitness studio, but *at-home workouts* can be just as effective in keeping you in shape, healthy, and fit, along with outdoors exercises that let you sweat "it" out while soaking up the sun (with your SPF of course!).

We provide you here with equipment-free exercises that get your heart pumping and the unwanted calories burning. These fitness routines allow you to sweat it out your way, on your own time, at your own place (or at the park).

Feel free to mix and match them depending on your health goals, capabilities, interests, and current physical condition.

> *1 hour workout is 4% of your day. No excuses.*
> —Anonymous

> *If you don't have time to warm up, you don't have time to work out.*
> —Nerdfitness.com

Doing warm-ups prior to any workout is critical for not only preventing injury but also for preparing your body and mind. A proper warm-up gets your blood, heart, lungs, muscles, your whole body, and your mindset ready for the more demanding part of your fitness routine: the main workout exercises.

Therefore, take the time to "warm yourself up" before you move on to the main and more intense set of the workout plan.

Quick Tip

Fitness routines vary in intensity and length, depending on the type of physical activity you do. According to the American Heart Association, warming up for five to ten minutes is ideal.

REGULAR, STATIC STRETCHING: IS IT A GOOD WARM-UP EXERCISE?

Static stretches involve no movement and require you to stay in one position for a period of time, normally somewhere between ten and sixty seconds per set. The typical "touch your toes" stretch is one example of static stretching.

Stretching a muscle in this way before any strenuous physical activity can increase the risk of injury from pulls and tears because it limits your body's ability to react quickly. Therefore, *avoid static stretching* for warm-ups and do it instead as your "after exercise" when your muscles are warm and flexible.

Instead, *do dynamic stretching* as a form of warm-up exercise because it incorporates active movement and moves your limbs through their full range of motion.

The following are some examples of dynamic stretching exercises: making shoulder circles, arm swings, side bends, hip circles and twist, leg swings, and squats.

QUICK AND EASY WARM-UP EXERCISE ROUTINE

You only need an exercise mat (or big towel), a timer, and your body. This warm-up routine is best for all types of workouts.

Do each exercise for 30 seconds with no pause. This is total of 5 minutes warm-up.

Walking High Knees + Backward Lunges + Squats + Inchworms + Hip Openers + Jumping Jacks + Arm Circles Forward + Arm Circles Backward

WALKING HIGH KNEES
- Stand straight and arms at your side and feet shoulder-width apart.
- Bring up your left knee above your belt line or as high as you can.
- Walk one step forward, lower your leg back down, and transition to the other leg.
- Repeat by lifting up the opposite knee toward your chest.
- *Carry on alternating back and forth while walking.*

BACKWARD LUNGES
- Stand straight and feet hips-width apart.
- Take one large step backward with your right foot, and lower your body toward the floor (right knee bent at a 90-degree angle).

- Pause for 2 seconds not touching the floor.
- Return and switch to your left leg.
  Inhale when you go down and exhale when you go up.
- Push through your front heel to go up.
- Return to start and repeat.

SQUATS
- Stand tall with your feet underneath your hips and shoulder-distance apart, and your toes forward.
- Sit all the way back (as if you're in a chair) and stand all the way up, nice and tall (make sure that your knees stay behind your toes).
- Rise back to start and repeat.

INCHWORMS
- Stand straight with your feet shoulder-width apart.
- Bend from your hips (legs straight) until your hands reach the floor and are as close as possible to your feet, allowing your back to bend forward.
- Walk your hands out one at a time and up until you're into a push-up position (core in straight line).
- Walk your hands back all the way to your feet (legs staying straight) and stand back up.
- Rise back to start and repeat.

HIP OPENERS
- Stand tall and straight and balance on your left leg.
- Lift your right knee up to waist height to meet your elbow.
- Open hip up to the right
  (Knee Motion: UP, OPEN, CENTER, DOWN).
- Switch to your left knee and then do "UP, OPEN, CENTER, DOWN" motion.
- Return and start to repeat switching from right to right and left to right.

JUMPING JACKS

- Stand upright and feet together and arms at your side.
- Bend your knees slightly, and jump up with your feet apart, arms stretched out and hands over your head (both legs out, both legs in).
- Jump back to starting position and repeat.

ARM CIRCLING

- Stand straight and feet shoulder-width apart.
- Take your arms up, parallel to the floor (extend your arms as far as you can).
- Move arms counterclockwise in small circles (arms straight, hands and palms down).
- Gradually go from small circles to big circles.
- Change direction and start circling your arms backward.
- Do at least 20 reps in each direction and as fast as you can.

15-MINUTE INDOOR BODY WEIGHT HIIT WORKOUT

High Intensity Interval Training, or *HIIT*, is a cardiovascular exercise strategy alternating short bursts of strenuous exercise with quick rest periods until you're too exhausted to continue.

For this 15-minute indoor bodyweight HIIT workout, we put together some of our favorite equipment-free and gym-less movements. They are challenging (as in all HIIT workouts), but you'll see visible results in no time if done correctly and regularly.

Perform each move for 45 seconds; rest 15 seconds after each move.

You need a mat, interval timer, your body, and a bottle of water to keep you hydrated.

Mountain Climbers + Squat Jacks + Leg Lifts + Skaters + Walking Lunges

MOUNTAIN CLIMBERS

The *mountain climbers* are a great total-body exercise and a go-to fitness routine that utilizes and activates your core.

This exercise improves your ability to strengthen and stabilize your spine and lower back. And because this exercise is usually performed with speed, it becomes an effective cardiovascular-type movement.

- Get down on the floor with your hands and knees getting into a plank position.
- Move your right leg toward the right hand, without lifting up your hips. (If flexibility is an issue, move the leg to whatever range is possible for you without the hips elevating.)
- Alternately move your legs back and forth (right leg close to right hand and left leg close to left hand), moving in and out nice and quickly.

Quick Tips

Keep your hands directly underneath your shoulder joint. Keep a straight line from wrist to elbow to shoulder. The hips should be right below your shoulders. Feet should be hip-width apart. Bring one knee toward your chest, one foot at a time.

SQUAT JACKS

The *squat jacks* are an effective cardio and legs exercise and work all your large muscle groups, especially your glutes. It's a go-to exercise for toning your glutes and thighs fast.

- Start standing with your feet close together and both hands by your side.
- Jump your feet up and simultaneously bend your knees so you land in a squat position.
- Push off using your heels and jump back up and return to the starting position.
- Repeat until 45 seconds is up.

Quick Tips

- Jump straight up with as much force as possible, but try to land softly on toes with your knees slightly bent.

- Put the force on your heels, jump back up, and breathe out as you do it.

LEG LIFTS / LEG RAISE

The *leg lift* is one of the best and simplest exercises to attain a flat belly.
- While it is a great abdominal movement, it has to be done right, otherwise you're barely working your abs (note: core strength is more important than getting a six-pack).
- Lay all the way down on your back, legs straight and together, with hands down by your side.
- Raise your legs off the ground and all the way up until they point at the ceiling. Keep them as straight as possible (toes pointed).
- Bring your legs back down until they're just a tiny bit above the ground. Hold them there for as long as you can.
- Lift your legs back up again. Repeat until you've done it or 45 seconds.

Quick Tips
- Avoid arching your lower back, so as not to let ab muscles slack off.
- Don't hurl your legs around until you are on solid ground, lying face up with arms at your sides and your legs extended.
- Press your lower back into the floor. Hold that for 15 seconds with your back pressed firmly into the floor.

SKATERS

The *skaters* are a cardiovascular exercise that shifts your body from side to side, creating a skating stride. It gets your heart rate up and helps a lot in slimming you down (if that's one of your goals). It strengthens your legs and improves your stability and balance.
- Bend left leg at a slight angle while maintaining weight and balance on the right leg.
- Raise your right leg out behind you, and swing your right hand toward your left foot.

- Leap sideways off your left foot and land on your right foot (with slightly bent hips and knees).
- As you leap, bring the left foot behind you and the left arm in front of you.
- Repeat the side-to-side motion in a skating-like movement. Do it for 3 sets or for 45 seconds.

Quick Tip
Don't lean forward too much (keep it to a 45-degree angle).

WALKING LUNGES
If you are keen on strengthening your leg muscles, as well as your core, hips, and glutes, the *walking lunge* is one of the best exercises that you can do. It improves your balance and core strength while simultaneously targeting your lower body's major muscle groups.
- Stand with your feet hip-width apart, hands on your hips or on the sides of your body.
- Move forward by taking a big step with your right leg and then getting down into a lunge position by bending your right knee at a 90-degree angle.
- Drive through your right foot to stand up out of the lunge.
- Repeat this movement alternating left and right legs until you've done it for 45 seconds.

Quick Tips
- If you don't have a whole lot of space, you can still do the lunge, moving forward and moving back, and if you have the space, you can walk all the way with it.
- You can make walking lunges more challenging by adding weights or doing a walking lunge with a torso twist.

JUMP YOUR WAY TO BETTER HEALTH!

Jump rope for 20 seconds and rest for 10 seconds. Repeat for 8 reps and do 3 sets.

Body Position: Hips over knees, shoulders over hips, chin down (for better air supply), head straight, abs up and in, with hips, shoulders, and knees low to the floor.

Arm Placement: Keep elbows in at your waist and your arms at a 90-degree angle (keep arms up and in).

Jumping Height: Nice and low to the ground.

Quick Tip

Size does matter when it comes to your skipping rope. So, get a rope that's appropriate for your height. To size your jump rope correctly, stand on the rope with your two feet together, then pull the handles up beside your body so the tops of the handles reach your armpits. That will be the correct size of your jump rope.

READY, SET, WALK!

Walk at a regular (comfortable) pace for 5–10 minutes and walk quickly for 1 minute. Return to a comfortable pace for 1 minute. Repeat the pattern for a total of 30 minutes (or more if this becomes too easy).

Alternatively, you may also just do a nice, long walk in the park (or anywhere safe) for an hour or two (or more)!

Proper Walking: Keep your head up, elongate your spine (avoid slouching), keep your shoulders down and back, engage your core (pull your belly button in toward your spine as you walk), swing your arms, and step from heel to toe.

Quick Tip

Walk better with flat, flexible athletic shoes that fit your feet perfectly right. Appreciate your walking environment and have fun!

JOG OFF THE POUNDS

Jog at a slow or moderate (comfortable) pace for 30 minutes a day (2–4 miles per run), 5 days a week, with a speed between 5 and 6 mph, and with high-enough intensity to raise your heart rate for at least several minutes. If you are breathing deeply but can still carry on a conversation (and can still smile), then you're doing well and not overstressing your body. *Proper Jogging:* Have a relaxed posture in your upper body. Keep your arms beside your body, and hold them in a 90-degree position. Land with a bent knee and your foot as close to flat as possible. Breathe regularly and smile.

Quick Tips

- Start off slow and easy on your first few jogs. Jog for 5 minutes, then walk for 2 minutes, and continue doing it like this for a while until your body is able to adjust and starts getting used to the workout.
- Invest in a good pair of jogging shoes.
- Do jog in place if the weather is not good and you need to work out at home.

OTHER "SWEAT IT OUT" EXERCISES

TAKE THE STAIRS!
This can be done at any place where there is a staircase (at home or in public places). It's more effective and beneficial for your fitness goals if you skip every other step. If you don't have a staircase at home, consider incorporating steps into your daily life. For example, you can use the stairs instead of the elevator in places where you have the option to use either. It can be a fun and easy way to sneak in a little body movement to your regular day.

CYCLE TO HEALTH!
If you're keen on a fitness routine that improves not only your physical health but also your emotional and mental well-being, *cycling is it!*

Outdoors, fresh air, and open space are always good for body, mind, and soul. Integrate these with a physical activity like cycling and you hit the healthy jackpot! You can ride solo, giving you "alone" time to reflect on *you*, or you can ride with a group to strengthen and broaden your social circle.

LET'S DANCE!
What can be more fun than dancing your way to fitness? Sweat away to your favorite dance moves. You can dance nice and slow, or you can do some heart-pounding, calorie-torching dance routine. Whatever suits you! The bottom line is you will have fun while staying fit and healthy.

SWIM YOUR WAY TO FITNESS!
Swimming gets your whole body moving without impacting your joints. So, swimming is especially a recommended exercise for those who suffer from joint pains (and arthritis).

It's important to note that when you swim, the water's buoyancy supports your body. In fact, 90 percent of your body weight is being supported by it; therefore, swimming places less stress on your joints.

You don't need to have your own swimming pool to do this. You can sign up for a public (or private) swimming club and join others. And yes, of course, you have to learn how to swim!

Important!

If you're in generally good health, can normally walk down a block, can run a quick errand to the market, and are not really a couch potato, you'll usually be fine to start with light to moderate physical activity without seeing your doctor.

However, if you've never had regular exercise for a prolonged period of time, plus you have a health condition or are at risk for certain medical problems, *please get your doctor's go-signal* before you start sprinting, running, mountain climbing, or doing any new fitness routine, especially if it's strenuous. Your physician can advise you in terms of how much exercise is safe for you considering your age, physical condition, medical history, and other key factors.

Starting an exercise program that is more intense than you are ready for can cause injury and serious medical issues.

A NOTE ABOUT WORKING OUT

ANY EXERCISE IS GOOD, BUT WHEN DONE RIGHT, exercise yields more substantial results (and injuries are minimized if not totally avoided). Here are *four thoughts to live by* when it comes to working out.

1. CONSISTENCY IS KEY.

This is a "nonnegotiable." It isn't the miles you've covered, the repetitions you've done; it's not even the physique you've got now, and it's certainly not your speed that matters most. Well, we all know the story of the Tortoise and the Hare. The Hare was thought to be the sure winner, but of course, the Tortoise surprisingly prevailed. All thanks to being steady (even if slow). The same goes for exercise.

To achieve consistency, you will want to think about the exercise routines that *you can and want to* do a few times a week, on a regular basis, for a prolonged period of time. It's also very helpful to have a workout plan that you will follow. If you want to know the best workout plan, well, it's actually any exercise you have fun (and love) doing and will do consistently.

2. INTENSITY MATTERS.

Any physical movement counts when it comes to staying fit and healthy, but you need to put in more effort for optimal health benefits.

The World Health Organization recommends that adults between the ages of eighteen and sixty-four do at least 150– 300 minutes of moderate-intensity aerobic exercise per week. It's important that you exercise hard enough without overstressing your body. Here's how to determine the intensity level of your exercise:

- *Low-Intensity Activities*
  You can talk and can still hum a song.

- *Moderate-Intensity Activities*
  You can converse but can't sing.
- *High-Intensity Activities*
  Speaking in full, coherent sentences is not possible.

For best results, you need to keep track of your heart rate and keep it above 60 percent and below 90 percent of your age-adjusted maximum. Here's how to calculate the range of your heart rate: *220 minus your age and then multiply it by 0.6 and 0.9.* For example, if your age is forty-five, 220 - 45 = 175 maximum heart rate 175 x 0.6 = 105 minimum training heart rate 175 x 0.9 = 157.5 maximum training rate

3. PROGRESSION RULES!

You've probably heard of this expression a lot of times, and that's because it's true. Progression of exercise refers to the process of increasing the intensity, duration, frequency, or amount of activity or exercise as the body adapts to a given activity pattern.

For aerobic exercise we have in this chapter, below is the ideal progression sequence: *Increase Duration* For example, increase duration of exercise session by 5 to 10 minutes every 1 to 2 weeks over the first 4 to 6 weeks. *Increase in Intensity and Frequency* For example, increase frequency and intensity of exercise session as tolerated over the next 4 to 8 months.

4. HAVE FUN!

Unless you have a very specific body build that you're trying to achieve, *any* physical movement is good news for your health and well-being. So, choose an exercise routine that you love, because if you love it, you'll have fun doing it and you'll keep doing it.

The fact is, exercise is only 10 percent of the health equation (90 percent is nutrition), and that's why there's no need to waste time doing an exercise you hate.

So, if you ever do it, enjoy it!

NOTES

(Journal articles are internet searchable using the DOI numbers. Other resources are internet searchable using the information provided.)

"About the Black Women's Health Study." Black Women's Health Study, Slone Epidemiology Center, Boston University. Available on the Boston University website.

Abe, R., N. Kumagai, M. Kimura, et al. "Biological Characteristics of Breast Cancer in Obesity." *Tohoku Journal of Experimental Medicine* 120, no. 4 (1976): 351–359. DOI: 10.1620/tjem.120.351.

Acheampong, Irene, and Lauren Haldeman. "Are Nutrition Knowledge, Attitudes, and Beliefs Associated with Obesity Among Low-Income Hispanic and African American Women Caretakers? *Journal of Obesity*. 2013. DOI: 10.1155/2013/123901.

"Accessory Breast Tissue." Radiopaedia. Updated 2024. Available online.

"Adjustment to Cancer: Anxiety, and Distress." National Cancer Institute, University of Pennsylvania. Oncolink.org, 2023. Available online.

"Adult Obesity Facts." Centers for Disease Control and Prevention. Updated 2022. Available online.

"Adult Obesity: A Global Look at Rising Obesity Rates." Harvard School of Public Health. Available on the Harvard University website.

Alsheik, N., L. Blount, Q. Qiong, et al. "Outcomes by Race in Breast Cancer Screening with Digital Breast Tomosynthesis Versus Digital Mammography." *Journal of the American College of Radiology* 18, no. 7 (2021): 906–918. DOI: 10.1016/j.jacr.2020.12.033.

Altomara, Deanna. "Breast Reduction Surgery: An Overview." WebMD. Reviewed 2023. Available online.

American College of Cardiology/American Heart Association Task Force on Practice Guidelines, Obesity Expert Panel. 2013. "Expert Panel Report: Guidelines (2013) for the Management of Overweight and Obesity in Adults." *Obesity (Silver Spring)* 22 (2014). Suppl 2: S41–410. DOI: 10.1002/oby.20660.

"Ancient Egypt: Ages 7–11." The British Museum. Available online.

Argolo, Daniel F., Clifford A. Hudis, and Neil M. Iyengar. "The Impact of Obesity on Breast Cancer." *Current Oncology Reports* 20 (2018). DOI: 10.1007/s11912-018-0688-8.

Aspan, Maria. "'We Can't Ever Go to the Doctor with Our Guard Down:' Why Black Women are 40% More Likely to Die of Breast Cancer." *MPW* (blog) by Fortune, 2020. Available online.

Assad, Hadeel, Gauri Badhwar, Sameeksha Bhama, et al. "Impact of Breast Cancer Diagnosis and Treatment on Sexual Dysfunction." Journal of Clinical Oncology 32 (2014). DOI: 10.1200/jco.2014.32.26_suppl.125.

Atoum, Manar, and Foad Alzoughool. "Vitamin D and Breast Cancer: Latest Evidence and Future Steps." *Breast Cancer: Basic and Clinical Research* 11 (2017). DOI: 10.1177/1178223417749816.

Bakyawa, Jennifer. "Uganda Fights Stigma, Poverty to Slay Breast Cancer Dragon." Nation, Kenya Edition 2013. Updated 2020. Available online.

Barber, Nigel. "Sexual Wiring of Women's Breasts." *Psychology Today*, 2013. Available online.

Behr, Tracy. "Finding a Lump in Breast Tissue." Breastfeeding Problems, 2021. Available online.

Berger, Ann M., Kathi Mooney, Amy Alvarez-Perez, et. al. "Caner-Related Fatigue, Version 2.2015." *Journal of the National Comprehensive Cancer Network* 13, no. 8 (2015): 1012–1039. DOI: 10.6004/jnccn.2015.0122.

Bhaskaran, Krishnan, Ian Douglas, Harriet Forbes, et al. "Body-Mass Index and Risk of 22 Specific Cancers: A Population-Based Cohort Study of 5.24 Million UK Adults." *Lancet* 384, no. 9945 (2014):755–765. DOI: 10.1016/S0140-6736(14)60892-8.

"'Billboard' Music Awards: Drake, Ye Win Big." DeltaPlex News, 2022. Available online.

"Black Women Added to High-Risk Group for Breast Cancer." Breastcancer.org, 2018. Available online.

Bolton, Elizabeth. "Imposter Syndrome from a Different Perspective: When Cancer and a Stroke Made Me Feel Like a fraud." Medium. Available online.

Bower, J. E., P. A. Ganz, K. A. Desmond, et al. "Fatigue in Breast Cancer Survivors: Occurrence, Correlates, and Impact on Quality of Life." *Journal of Clinical Oncology* 18, no. 4 (2000): 743–753. DOI: 10.1200/JCO.2000.18.4.743.

"BWHS Researchers Develop Breast Cancer Prediction Tool for Black Women." Black Women's Health Study, Slone Epidemiology Center, Boston University, 2021. Available on the Boston University website.

"Breast Augmentation." American Society of Plastic Surgeons, 2021. Available online.

"Breast Cancer: Breast Cancer is the Most Diagnosed Cancer Globally." Union for International Cancer Control, 2023. Available online.

"Breast Cancer Facts & Figures 2022–2024." American Cancer Society, 2022. Available online.

"Breast Cancer and Intimacy." SurvivingBreastCancer.org. Available online.

"Breast Cancer Myths." National Breast Cancer Foundation. Available online.

"Breast Cancer Risk: Body Weight and Weight Gain." Susan G. Komen. Updated 2023. Available online.

"Breast Cancer Risk and Prevention." American Cancer Society, 2021. Available online.

"Breast Cancer Screening." NIH National Cancer Institute Cancer Trends Progress Report. Updated 2023. Available online.

"Breast Cancer Statistics and Resources." Breast Cancer Research Foundation. Available online.

"Breast Cancer Treatment (PDQ®)–Patient Version." National Cancer Institute, NIH. Updated 2023. Available online.

"Breast Density and Your Mammogram Report." American Cancer Society. Updated 2023. Available online.

"Breast Feeding and Breast Engorgement." Drugs.com. Updated 2023. Available online.

Breast Form Model 356: Essential Light. Amoena. Available for sale online on womanspersonalhealth.com.

"Breast Imaging Reporting & Data System (BI-RADS)." Atlas, 5th edition (2013). Website contains free information. American College of Radiology.

"Breast Implants." U.S. Food and Drug Administration, 2023. Available online.

"Breast Pain." Mayo Clinic, 2023. Available online.

"Breast Self-Exam." BreastCancer.org. Available online.

"Breasts." Bible Doctrine News (definition). Available online.

Bu, Xiaofan, Shuangshuang Li, Andy S. K. Cheng, et al. "Breast Cancer Stigma Scale: A Reliable and Valid Stigma Measure for Patients with Breast Cancer." *Frontiers in Psychology* 13 (2022). DOI: 10.3389/fpsyg.2022.841280.

Bucher, Meg. "5 Life-Changing Ways to Keep Faith Over Fear." Crosswalk, 2020. Available online.

Bulletin des lois de la République française (Bulletin of the Laws of the French Republic). Entry for Cadolle's *corselet-gorge*, the first bra, 1900. Available on the Gallica website.

CA: A Cancer Journal for Clinicians. The American Cancer Society. Available online.

Calle, Eugenia E., Carmen Rodriguez, Kimberly Walker-Thurmond, et al. "Overweight, Obesity, and Mortality from Cancer in a Prospectively Studied Cohort of U.S. Adults." *New England Journal of Medicine* 348, no. 17 (2003):1625–1638. DOI: 10.1056/NEJMoa021423.

"Cancer Attributable to Obesity." Analysis tools; International Agency for Research on Cancer. Available on the gco.iarc.fr website.

"Cancer Stigma and Silence Around the World: A LiveStrong Report." LiveStrong. Available online.

"Cancer Today: Top Cancer per Country, Estimated Number of Deaths in 2020, Females, All Ages (Excl. NMSC)." International Agency for Research on Cancer. Available on the gco.iarc.fr website.

Carter, Devon. "3 Things to Know About Breast Cancer Survivorship." M. D. Anderson Center, University of Texas, October 28, 2020. Available on the *Cancerwise* blog.

Chaturvedi, Santosh K. Psychiatric Oncology: Cancer in Mind. *Indian Journal of Psychiatry* 54, no. 2 (2012): 111–118. DOI: 10.4103/0019-5545.99529.

Chen, Peizhan, Pingting Hu, Dong Xie, et al. "Meta-analysis of vitamin D, calcium and the prevention of breast cancer." *Breast Cancer Research and Treatment* 121, no. 2 (2010): 469–477. DOI: 10.1007/s10549-009-0593-9.

"Common Breast Cancer-Related Fears." BreastCancer.org. Updated 2022. Available online.

"Common Breast Problems." Women's Health Clinic. Available online.

"Complementary and Alternative Medicine." National Cancer Institute, NIH. Updated 2023. Available online.

"Complementary and Integrative Medicine." American Academy of Child & Adolescent Psychiatry, 2017. Available online.

"Cooling Caps (Scalp Hypothermia) to Reduce Hair Loss." American Cancer Society. Updated 2022. Available online.

"Dense Breast Q&A Guide." National Breast Cancer Foundation, Inc. Updated 2024. Available online.

DePolo, Jamie. "Cancerous Phyllodes Tumors of the Breast." Breastcancer.org, 2023. Available online.

Doyle, Chase. "Treating Sexual Dysfunction in Breast Cancer Survivors." *Journal of Oncology & Navigation Survivorship* 6, no. 6 (2015). Available online.

Duran, Alexandra. "History of the Bra." *Women's Health*. Available online.

Edelen, Maria Orlando, Anita Chandra, Brian Stucky, et al. "Developing a Global Cancer Stigma Index." *SAGE Open* 4, no. 3 (2014). DOI: 10.1177/2158244014547875.

Eke, Onyinyechi, Onyeka Otugo, and Jessica Isom. "Black Women in Medicine—Rising Above Invisibility." *The Lancet* 397, no. 10,274 (2021): 573–574. Available online.

Elreda, Lauren, Angelina Kim, and Manmeet Malik. "Mitigating Breast Cancer Disparities by Addressing the Obesity Epidemic." *Current Breast Cancer Reports* 14 (2022): 168–173. DOI: 10.1007/s12609-022-00460-4.

Esserman, Laura, and Beth Crawford. "You Don't Have to Fear Breast Cancer." CNN Health, 2013. Available online.

"Exploring the Potential Benefits of Cannabidiol (CBD) for Health and Wellness." Available on the Healthopedia UK website.

Fayanju, Oluwadamilola M., Susan Kraenzle, Bettina F. Drake, et al. "Perceived Barriers to Mammography Among Underserved Women in a Breast Health Center Outreach Program. *The American Journal of Surgery* 208, no. 3 (2014): 425–434. DOI: 10.1016/j.amjsurg.2014.03.005.

"Fighting Stigma & Poverty Related to Breast Cancer in Uganda." UICC.org. Updated 2019. Available online.

Finnigan, Kate. "Soft Focus: The New Lingerie Evolution. *Financial Times*, 2020. Available online.

Fiorentino, Lavinia and Sonia Ancoli-Israel. "Insomnia and Its Treatment in Women with Breast Cancer." *Sleep Medicine Reviews* 10, no. 6(2006): 419–429. DOI: 10.1016/j.smrv.2006.03.005.

Fiorentino, Lavinia, Michelle Rissling, Lianqi Liu, et al. "The Symptom Cluster of Sleep, Fatigue and Depressive Symptoms in Breast Cancer Patients: Severity of the Problem and Treatment Options." *Drug Discovery Today: Disease Models* 8, no. 4 (2011): 167–173. DOI: 10.1016/j.ddmod.2011.05.001.

Flowers, Chris I., Blaise P. Mooney, and Jennifer S. Drukteinis. *Clinical and Imaging Surveillance Following Breast Cancer Diagnosis*. American Society of Clinical Oncology Educational Book, vol. 32, 2012. DOI: 10.14694/EdBook_AM.2012.32.220.

"Food List." Eat to Beat Cancer: Universal Health Atlas. Available online.

Frette, Juliette. "The Meaning of Breasts." Huffpost, 2011. Available online.

Fryberg, Stephanie A., and Sarah S. M. Townsend. "The Psychology of Invisibility." In G. Adams, et al. (editors.), *Commemorating Brown: The Social Psychology of Racism and Discrimination* 2008 (173–193). American Psychological Association. DOI: 10.1037/11681-010.

Galukande, M., J. Schüz, B. O. Anderson, et al. "Maternally Orphaned Children and Intergenerational Concerns Associated with Breast Cancer Deaths Among Women in Sub-Saharan Africa." *JAMA Oncology* 7, no. 2 (2021): 285–289. DOI: 10.1001/jamaoncol.2020.6583.

Ganz, Patricia A., Lorna Kwan, Annette L. Stanton, et al. "Physical and Psychosocial Recovery in the Year After Primary Treatment of Breast Cancer."

Journal of Clinical Oncology 29, no. 9 (2011): 1101–1109. DOI: 10.1200/JCO.2010.28.8043.

Garrity-Bond, Cynthie. "The Tale of Two Breast: From Religious Symbol to Secular Object." Feminism and Religion, 2012. Available online.

Gillespie, Tessa C., Hoda E. Sayegh, Cheryl L.Brunelle, et al. "Breast Cancer-Related Lymphedema: Risk Factors, Precautionary Measures, and Treatments." *Gland Surgery* 7, no. 4 (2018): 379–403. DOI: 10.21037/gs.2017.11.04.

"The Global Cancer Stigma Index." LiveStrong Foundation, 2011. Available online.

"Global Survey 2020." The International Society of Aesthetic Plastic Surgery, 2020. Available on the ISAPS.org website.

Go Ask Alice! Columbia University (health question database: search "breasts). Available online.

Goffman E. *Stigma: Notes on the Management of Spoiled Identity*. Englewood Cliffs: Prentice Hall, 1963.

Grady, Denise. "Uganda Fights Stigma and Poverty to Take on Breast Cancer." *New York Times*, 2013.

Hailu, Haimanot E., Alison M. Mondul, Laura S. Rozek, et al. "Descriptive Epidemiology of Breast and Gynecological Cancers Among Patients Attending St. Paul's Hospital Millennium Medical College, Ethiopia." *PLOS One* 15, no. 3 (2020), e0230625. DOI: 10.1371/journal.pone.0230625.

HairToStay. A 501c3 nonprofit organization that helps low-income cancer patients afford scalp cooling treatment. Information available online.

Hamel, P. J. "My Story." *Dartmouth Medicine*, spring 2009. Dartmouth College. Available on the Dartmouth College website.

Hamilton, Laura. Quoted by Liesha Getson in the October newsletter (n.d.). Thermographic and Diagnostic Imaging and Health Through Awareness. Available online.

Hermann, Francoise. "Oh, Patents! The Corset-Bra (1898)." Patents on the Soles of Your Shoes (blog), 2017. Available online.

Hsu, Tina, Marguerite Ennis, Nicky Hood, et al. "Quality of Life in Long-Term Breast Cancer Survivors." *Journal of Clinical Oncology* 31, no. 28 (2013): 3540–3548.

"Is Cancer Treatment Affecting Your Skin and Nails?" Health Essentials, Cleveland Clinic, 2021. Available online.

Jang, Andrew, Chris Brown, Gillian Lamoury, et al. "The Effects of Acupuncture on Cancer-Related Fatigue: Updated Systematic Review and Meta-Analysis." *Integrative Cancer Therapies* 19 (2020). DOI: 10.1177/1534735420949679.

Jiralerspong, Sao, and Pamela Goodwin. "Obesity and Breast Cancer Prognosis: Evidence, Challenges, and Opportunities." *Journal of Clinical Oncology* 34, no. 35 (2016): 4203–4216. DOI: 10.1200/JCO.2016.68.4480.

Johnson, Veronica R., Nonyerem O. Acholonu, Ana C. Dolan, et al. *Current Obesity Reports* 10, no. 3 (2021): 342–350. DOI: 10.1007/s13679-021-00442-0.

Joly, Florence, Marie Lange, Melanie Dos Santos, et al. "Long-Term Fatigue and Cognitive Disorders in Breast Cancer Survivors" *Cancers* 11, no. 12 (2019). DOI: 10.3390/cancers11121896.

Journal of Breast Imaging. The Society of Breast Imaging. Searchable online using PubMed.

Keyser, Erin A., Barton C. Staat, Merlin B. Fausett, et al. "Pregnancy-Associated Breast Cancer." *Reviews in Obstetrics & Gynecology* 5, no. 2 (2012): 94–99.

King, Martin Luther. "What Is Your Life's Blueprint?" Speech; Philadelphia, October 26, 1967. Available on *The Seattle Times* website.

Koehler, L. A., T. C. Haddad, D. W. Hunter, et al. "Axillary Web Syndrome Following Breast Cancer Surgery: Symptoms, Complications, And Management Strategies." *Breast Cancer* 11 (2019): 13–19. DOI: 10.2147/BCTT.S146635.

Lam, Diana L., Nehmat Houssami, and Janie M. Lee. "Imaging Surveillance After Primary Breast Cancer Treatment." *American Journal of Roentgenology* 208, no. 3 (2017). DOI: 10.2214/AJR.16.16300.

Lauby-Secretan, Beatrice, Chiara Scoccianti, Dana Loomis, et al. "Body Fatness and Cancer—Viewpoint of the IARC Working Group." *New England Journal of Medicine* 375, no. 8 (2016): 794–798. DOI: 10.1056/NEJMsr1606602.

Lee, Kyuwan, Laura Kruper, Christina M. Dieli-Conwright, et al. "The Impact of Obesity on Breast Cancer Diagnosis and Treatment." *Current Oncology Reports* 21 (2019). DOI: 10.1007/s11912-019-0787-1.

Living Beyond Breast Cancer Blog: Real People Sharing Real-Life Experiences About Real Issues to Educate, Motivate, and Inspire You. Available online.

Living Beyond Breast Cancer: Downloads (free information). Available online.

"Living as a Breast Cancer Survivor." American Cancer Society. Available online.

Love, Susan M. *Dr. Susan Love's Breast Book*, 7th ed. Hachette, New York: 2023.

"Mammogram Basics." American Cancer Society, 2022. Available online.

"Mammograms." American Cancer Society, 2022. Available online.

McLean, Nicole. "Handling Feelings of Being a Fraud." Fabulous Boobies (blog), 2014. Available online.

Miles, Margaret R. *A Complex Delight: The Secularization of the Breast, 1350–1750*. University of California Press, Berkeley: 2008.

Momoh, Adeyiza O., Aisha J. McKnight, Anthony Echo, et al. "The First Silicone Breast Implant Patient: A 47-Year Follow-Up." *Plastic and Reconstructive Surgery* 125, no. 6 (2010): 226e–229e. DOI: 10.1097/PRS.0b013e3181d180d0.

"Most Valuable Bra: Heavenly Star Bra by Victoria's Secret." Guinness World Records, 2024. Available online.

Munteanu, Carmen. "History of Breast Implants and Origins of Breast Enlargement Surgery." Aesthetik Profile, 2021. Available online.

Murray, Donna. "Breastfeeding with Small Breasts." Verywell Family, 2021. Available online.

Murray, Donna. "How Breast Size and Shape Affects Breastfeeding." Verywell Family, 2021. Available online.

"National Cancer Survivorship Resource Center." American Cancer Society. Available online.

NCCN Guidelines for Patients. "Survivorship Care for Cancer-Related Late and Long-Term Effects," 2020. Available online.

Neff, Kristin. Self-Compassion, 2024. Available online.

"*New York Times* Examines Breast Cancer in Uganda." 2013. Available on the KFF.org website.

"Normal Breast Development and Changes." Johns Hopkins Medicine. Available online.

"Obesity and Cancer Fact Sheet." National Cancer Institute, NIH, 2022. Available online.

OncoLife Survivorship Care Plan. University of Pennsylvania, Oncolink.org, 2023. Available online.

Orenstein, Peggy. "Our Feel-Good War on Breast Cancer." *New York Times Magazine*, 2013. Available online.

"Our History." Cadolle, lingerie company and inventor of the bra. Available online.

"Overcoming the Fear of Breast Cancer." HealthyWomen, 2014. Available online.

Pamula, Hanna. Flight Radiation Calculator. Omni Calculator, 2023. Available online.

Pappas, Stephanie, and Natalie Wolchover. "New Theory on Why Men Love Breasts." LiveScience, 2016. Available online.

Pedersen, Rikke Nørgaard, Buket Öztürk Esen, Lene Mellemkjær, et al. "The Incidence of Breast Cancer Recurrence 10–32 Years After Primary Diagnosis." *Journal of the National Cancer Institute* 114, no. 3 (2022): 391–399. DOI: 10.1093/jnci/djab202.

Perez, Frances, Ashley Bragg, and Gary Whitman. "Pregnancy Associated Breast Cancer." *Journal of Clinical Imaging Science* 11, no. 49 (2021). DOI: 10.25259/JCIS_81_2021.

Pfeffer, Jennifer. "21 Healthy Lifestyle Quotes to Inspire You." Jim Rohn quotation. Health and Wellness Blog, University of Rasmussen. Available online.

Phalak, Kanchan A., Emily L. Sedgwick, Sagar Dhamne, et al. "AIRP Best Cases in Radiologic-Pathologic Correlation: Malignant Phyllodes Tumor with Osteosarcomatous Differentiation." *RadioGraphics* 33, no. 5 (2013): 1377–1381. DOI: 10.1148/rg.335135004.

Phelan, S. M., D. J. Burgess, M. W. Yeazel, et al. "Impact of Weight Bias and Stigma on Quality of Care and Outcomes for Patients with Obesity." *Obesity Reviews* 16, no. 4 (2015): 319–326. DOI: 10.1111/obr.12266.

"Planning and Visualization Lead to Better Food Habits." McGill University, 2011. Available on the McGill University website.

Post, Lanneke, and Anke I. Liefbroer. "Reducing Distress in Cancer Patients: A Preliminary Evaluation of Short-Term Coaching by Expert Volunteers." *Psychooncology* 28, no. 8 (2019): 1762–1766. DOI: 10.1002/pon.5111.

Protani, Melinda, Michael Coory, and Jennifer H. Martin. "Effect of Obesity on Survival of Women with Breast Cancer: Systematic Review and Meta-Analysis. *Breast Cancer Research and Treatment* 123, no. 3 (2010): 627–635. DOI: 10.1007/s10549-010-0990-0.

Purdie-Vaughns, Valerie, and Richard P. Eibach. "Intersectional Invisibility: The Distinctive Advantages and Disadvantages of Multiple Subordinate-Group Identities." *Sex Roles: A Journal of Research* 59, no. 5–6 (2008): 377–391. DOI: 10.1007/s11199-008-9424-4.

"Radiation from Air Travel." Centers for Disease Control and Prevention, 2015. Available online.

Romieu, Isabelle, Laure Dossus, and Walter C. Willett (Eds.). *Energy Balance and Obesity*. IARC Working Group Reports Vol. 10. International Agency for Research on Cancer. World Health Organization, 2017. Available online.

Runowicz, Carolyn D., Corinne R. Leach, N. Lynn Henry, et al. "American Cancer Society/American Society of Clinical Oncology Breast Cancer Survivorship Care Guideline." *CA: A Cancer Journal for Clinicians* 66, no. 1 (2016): 43–73. DOI: 10.3322/caac.21319.

Sacks, Tina K. *Invisible Visits: Black Middle-Class Women in the American Healthcare System*. Oxford, Oxford University Press, 2019.

Sam, Kenny Q., Frederick J. Severs, Lilian O. Ebuoma, et al. "Granulomatous Mastitis in a Transgender Patient." *The Journal of Radiology Case Reports* 11, no. 2 (2017): 16–22. DOI: 10.3941/jrcr.v11i2.2934.

Saslow, Debbie, Carla Boetes, Wylie Burke, et al. "American Cancer Society guidelines for breast screening with MRI as an adjunct to mammography." *CA: A Cancer Journal for Clinicians* 57, no. 2 (2007): 75–89. DOI: 10.3322/canjclin.57.2.75.

Saul, Stephanie. "U.S. Ends Ban on Silicone Breast Implants." *New York Times*, 2006.

Schover, Leslie. "Will2Love: A New Resource to Improve Women's Sex Lives After Breast Cancer." Living Beyond Breast Cancer (blog) 2017. Available online.

Schwartz, John. "Dow Corning Accepts Implant Settlement Plan." *The Washington Post*, 1998.

Sesko, Amanda K., and Monica Biernat. "Prototypes of Race and Gender: The Invisibility of Black Women." *Journal of Experimental Social Psychology* 46, no. 2 (2010): 356–360.

Sheppard, Vanessa B., Jennifer Hicks, Kepher Makambi, et al. "The Feasibility and Acceptability of a Diet and Exercise Trial in Overweight and Obese Black Breast Cancer Survivors: The Stepping STONE Study. *Contemporary Clinical Trials* 46 (2016): 106–113. DOI: 10.1016/j.cct.2015.12.005.

The Sidney Kimmel Comprehensive Cancer Center. Johns Hopkins Medicine. Baltimore, MD. Information available online.

"Signs and Symptoms of Breast Cancer." BreastCancer.org. Updated 2023. Available online.

"State Law Map: Dense Breast Info." DenseBreast-info.org. Updated 2024. Available online.

"Study Finds Losing Weight After 50 May Lower Breast Cancer Risk." American Cancer Society, 2019. Available online.

Sulemann, B. B. M., C. van Dooijeweert, E. van der Wall, et al. "Pregnancy-Associated Breast Cancer: Nationwide Dutch Study Confirms a Discriminatory Aggressive Histopathologic Profile." *Breast Cancer Research and Treatment* 186, (2021): 699–704. DOI: 10.1007/s10549-021-06130-w.

Sung, H., J. Ferlay, R. L. Siegel, et al. "Global Cancer Statistics 2020: GLOBOCAN Estimates of Incidence and Mortality Worldwide for 36 Cancers in 185 Countries." *CA: A Cancer Journal for Clinicians* 71, no. 3 (2021): 209–249. DOI: 10.3322/caac.21660.

SurvivingBreastCancer.org. Breast Cancer News, Articles, Stories, and More!" (Blog) Available online.

Swinnen, Jeroen, Machteld Keupers, Julie Soens, et al. Breast Imaging Surveillance after Curative Treatment for Primary Non-Metastasised Breast Cancer in Non-High-Risk Women: A Systematic Review. *Insights into Imaging* 9, no. 6 (2018): 961–970. DOI: 10.1007/s13244-018-0667-5.

Teras, Lauren R., Alpa V. Patel, Molin Wang, et al. "Sustained Weight Loss and Risk of Breast Cancer in Women 50 Years and Older: A Pooled Analysis of Prospective Data." *Journal of the National Cancer Institute* 112, no. 9 (2020): 929–937. DOI: 10.1093/jnci/djz226.

Thompson, Paige. "The Relationship of Fatigue and Meaning in Life in Breast Cancer Survivors." *Oncology Nursing Forum* 34, no. 3 (2007): 653–660. DOI: 10.1188/07.ONF.653-660.

"Timeline: A Short History of Breast Implants." Reuters, 2012. Available online.

Torres-Lacomba, M., V. Prieto-Gómez, B. Arranz-Martín, et al. "Manual Lymph Drainage with Progressive Arm Exercises for Axillary Web Syndrome After Breast Cancer Surgery: A Randomized Controlled Trial." *Physical Therapy* 102, no. 3 (2022). DOI: 10.1093/ptj/pzab314.

"Treatment Options: Surgery." Breastcancer.org, 2024. Available online.

Tripathi L., S. S. Datta, S. K. Agrawal, et al. "Stigma Perceived by Women Following Surgery for Breast Cancer." Indian Journal of Medical and Paediatric Oncology. 38, no. 2 (2017): 146–152. DOI: 10.4103/ijmpo.ijmpo_74_16.

Uscher, Jen. "Cold Caps and Scalp Cooling Systems." Breastcancer.org. Updated 2023. Available online.

van Beek, Florie E., Lonneke M. A. Wijnhoven, Femke Jansen, et al. "Prevalence of Adjustment Disorder Among Cancer Patients, and the Reach, Effectiveness, Cost-Utility and Budget Impact of Tailored Psychological Treatment: Study Protocol of a Randomized Controlled Trial. *BMC Psychology* 7, article number 89 (2019). DOI: 10.1186/s40359-019-0368-y.

"Vitamin D and Breast Cancer: Is there a Connection?" Blackdoctor.org. Available online.

Wagstaff, Anna. "Stigma: Breaking the Vicious Cycle." *Cancerworld* 55 (2013). Available online.

"The Weird, Wild Legal History of Breasts and Nipples." Yahoo Health, 2014. Available online.

"What is Cancer Rehabilitation?" Cancer.net, American Society of Clinical Oncology. 2022. Available online.

"What is Lymphedema?" National Lymphedema Network. Available online.

"What to Know About Breast Implants." U.S. Food and Drug Administration, 2023. Available online.

Whitelocks, Sadie. "Photo of Breast Cancer Survivor's Tattooed Chest is Shared by Thousands after Facebook's Attempts to Ban it." Daily Mail, 2013. Available online.

Wijnhoven, Lonneke M. A., José A. E. Custers, Linda Kwakkenbos, et al. "Trajectories of Adjustment Disorder Symptoms in Post-Treatment Breast Cancer Survivors." Supportive Care in Cancer 30 (2022): 3521–3530. DOI: 10.1007/s00520-022-06806-z.

"The World's Most Popular Plastic Surgery Procedures." Pacific Heights Plastic Surgery, 2021. Available online.

Yoon, Jung Hyun, Min Jung Kim, Eun-Kyung Kim, et al. "Imaging Surveillance of Patients with Breast Cancer After Primary Treatment: Current Recommendations." *Korean Journal of Radiology*, 16, no. 2 (2015): 219–228. DOI: 10.3348/kjr.2015.16.2.2192015.

Zessin, Ulli, Oliver Dickhauser, and Sven Garbade. "The Relationship Between Self-Compassion and Well-Being: A Meta-Analysis." *Health and Well-Being* 7, no. 3, (2015): 340–364. DOI: 10.1111/aphw.12051.

"22 Myths and Truths." National Breast Cancer Coalition. Available online.

IMAGE CREDITS

SHUTTERSTOCK:

©Alex Hliv, ©pp_watchar, ©X-CT, ©Radiological Imaging, ©Xray Computer, ©PeopleImages.com - Yuri A, ©Antonina Vlasova, ©Lucky Business, ©Ilia Nesolenyi, ©zefirchik06, ©Yuliya Gontar, ©zi3000, ©Irina Neretina, ©Brent Hofacker, ©Wartiaja, ©Dream79, ©Timolina, ©mpephotos, ©zi3000, ©Anton27, ©Yevgeniya Shal, ©Svetlana Monyakova, ©from my point of view, ©Erhan Inga, ©Kyriakos, ©Timolina, ©5PH, ©Elena Schweitzer, ©Alphonsine Sabine, ©Foxys Forest Manufacture, ©Igor Normann, ©denio109, ©Tatiana Bralnina

ACKNOWLEDGEMENT

TO MY FAMILY, FRIENDS, MENTORS, colleagues, team members, and well-wishers—thank you for standing by me and fueling my passion. Your unwavering support has been the foundation of this book and mission, which is deeply rooted in love, empowerment, and our shared responsibility for the well-being of women.

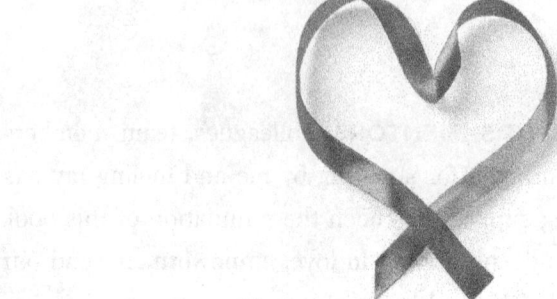

www.ingramcontent.com/pod-product-compliance
Lightning Source LLC
Chambersburg PA
CBHW020538030426
42337CB00013B/893